BODY LANGUAGE

Talk that Talk

Chase DuQuesnay EnQi ReaL

The Few....

CONTENTS

INTRODUCTION

This book has a couple of purposes, helping to develop teachers through writing and helping people feel more comfortable with **"Doctorese"**...

The syllabus is very simple for our developing Literians: patreon classes and assessments for each book that we have or the more specifically the subject matter therein...

Please read or reread the introduction to the PHD book, we intend to crush those goals! Each assessment you take, will be in essay form, this means that each essay can also be used, as a chapter in your book! This is a radically new type of "health" course...

Wordsmiths, Articulators, Literarians, Orthographers, Scribes & Lexicographers is our aim! We want you to build your mind, help others to build their mind, studying the body and mind. That is our Polyibic thing...

and yes... I still have 1 on 1 tuturing classes available in AmericanHealer.Website

THE OATH

ὄμνυμι Ἀπόλλωνα ἰητρὸν καὶ Ἀσκληπιὸν καὶ Ὑγείαν καὶ Πανάκειαν καὶ θεοὺς πάντας τε καὶ πάσας, ἵστορας ποιεύμενος, ἐπιτελέα ποιήσειν κατὰ δύναμιν καὶ κρίσιν ἐμὴν ὅρκον τόνδε καὶ συγγραφὴν τήνδε:
ἡγήσεσθαι μὲν τὸν διδάξαντά με τὴν τέχνην ταύτην ἴσα γενέτῃσιν ἐμοῖς, καὶ βίου κοινώσεσθαι, καὶ χρεῶν χρηΐζοντι μετάδοσιν ποιήσεσθαι, καὶ γένος τὸ ἐξ αὐτοῦ ἀδελφοῖς ἴσον ἐπικρινεῖν ἄρρεσι, καὶ διδάξειν τὴν τέχνην ταύτην, ἢν χρηΐζωσι μανθάνειν, ἄνευ μισθοῦ καὶ συγγραφῆς, παραγγελίης τε καὶ ἀκροήσιος καὶ τῆς λοίπης ἀπάσης μαθήσιος μετάδοσιν ποιήσεσθαι υἱοῖς τε ἐμοῖς καὶ τοῖς τοῦ ἐμὲ διδάξαντος, καὶ μαθητῇσι συγγεγραμμένοις τε καὶ ὡρκισμένοις νόμῳ ἰητρικῷ, ἄλλῳ δὲ οὐδενί.
διαιτήμασί τε χρήσομαι ἐπ᾿ ὠφελείῃ καμνόντων κατὰ δύναμιν καὶ κρίσιν ἐμήν, ἐπὶ δηλήσει δὲ καὶ ἀδικίῃ εἴρξειν.
οὐ δώσω δὲ οὐδὲ φάρμακον οὐδενὶ αἰτηθεὶς θανάσιμον, οὐδὲ ὑφηγήσομαι συμβουλίην τοιήνδε: ὁμοίως δὲ οὐδὲ γυναικὶ πεσσὸν φθόριον δώσω.
ἁγνῶς δὲ καὶ ὁσίως διατηρήσω βίον τὸν ἐμὸν καὶ τέχνην τὴν ἐμήν.
οὐ τεμέω δὲ οὐδὲ μὴν λιθιῶντας, ἐκχωρήσω δὲ ἐργάτῃσιν ἀνδράσι πρήξιος τῆσδε.
ἐς οἰκίας δὲ ὁκόσας ἂν ἐσίω, ἐσελεύσομαι ἐπ᾿ ὠφελείῃ καμνόντων, ἐκτὸς ἐὼν πάσης ἀδικίης ἑκουσίης καὶ φθορίης, τῆς τε ἄλλης καὶ ἀφροδισίων ἔργων ἐπί τε γυναικείων σωμάτων καὶ ἀνδρῴων, ἐλευθέρων τε καὶ δούλων.
ἃ δ᾿ ἂν ἐνθεραπείῃ ἴδω ἢ ἀκούσω, ἢ καὶ ἄνευ θεραπείης κατὰ βίον

ἀνθρώπων, ἃ μὴ χρή ποτε ἐκλαλεῖσθαι ἔξω, σιγήσομαι, ἄρρητα ἡγεύμενος εἶναι τὰ τοιαῦτα.
ὅρκον μὲν οὖν μοι τόνδε ἐπιτελέα ποιέοντι, καὶ μὴ συγχέοντι, εἴη ἐπαύρασθαι καὶ βίου καὶ τέχνης δοξαζομένῳ παρὰ πᾶσιν ἀνθρώποις ἐς τὸν αἰεὶ χρόνον· παραβαίνοντι δὲ καὶ ἐπιορκέοντι, τἀναντία τούτων.

I swear by Apollo Healer, by Asclepius, by Hygieia, by Panacea, and by all the gods and goddesses, making them my witnesses, that I will carry out, according to my ability and judgment, this oath and this indenture.

To hold my teacher in this art equal to my own parents; to make him partner in my livelihood; when he is in need of money to share mine with him; to consider his family as my own brothers, and to teach them this art, if they want to learn it, without fee or indenture; to impart precept, oral instruction, and all other instruction to my own sons, the sons of my teacher, and to indentured pupils who have taken the Healer's oath, but to nobody else.

I will use those dietary regimens which will benefit my patients according to my greatest ability and judgment, and I will do no harm or injustice to them. Neither will I administer a poison to anybody when asked to do so, nor will I suggest such a course. Similarly I will not give to a woman a pessary to cause abortion. But I will keep pure and holy both my life and my art. I will not use the knife, not even, verily, on sufferers from stone, but I will give place to such as are craftsmen therein.

Into whatsoever houses I enter, I will enter to help the sick, and I will abstain from all intentional wrong-doing and harm, especially from abusing the bodies of man or woman, bond or free. And whatsoever I shall see or hear in the course of my profession, as well as outside my profession in my intercourse with men, if it be what should not be published abroad, I will never divulge, holding such things to be holy secrets.

Now if I carry out this oath, and break it not, may I gain for ever reputation among all men for my life and for my art; but if I break it and forswear myself, may the opposite befall me.

SPANISH

Questions

- ¡Es una emergencia! – It's an emergency!
- Tenemos una emergencia. – We have an emergency.
- He tenido un accidente. – I've had an accident.
- ¿Tiene dolor? – Do you have pain?
- ¿Dónde le duele? – Where does it hurt?
- Me duele aquí. – It hurts here (Remember to point at the exact place where it hurts).
- ¿Quién es su contacto de emergencia? – Who is your emergency contact?
- ¿Qué medicinas toma? – Which medicines are you taking?
- ¿Está embarazada? – Are you pregnant?
- ¿Qué enfermedades o síntomas tiene, de que sepa usted? a) Ninguna b) Diabetes c) Del corazón d) De los pulmones e) De los riñones f) Úlceras g) Presión alta h) Convulsiones i) Artritis – What diseases or medical conditions do you have that you know about? a) None b) Diabetes c) Heart d) Lungs e) Kidneys f) Ulcer g) High blood pressure h) Seizures i) Arthritis
- **Puedo ayudarle** - can i help you
- **Ayúdame** - Help me
- **¿Tienes copago?** - do you have copay
- **¿Qué está cubierto por Medicaid?** - whats covered under medicaid
- **¿Tienes traductora/traductor?** - DO YOU HAVE A TRANSLATOR

Responses

- Tengo dolor. – I have pain/It hurts.
- Tengo dolor de… cabeza/ estómago/ garganta/ oídos/ muelas. – I have a… headache/ stomach ache/ sore throat/ sore ears/ tooth ache.
- Me duele… el brazo/ la pierna/ la rodilla/ el pie/ los dedos/ el tobillo/ el hombro/ la espalda/ la muñeca. – My arm/ leg/ knee/ foot/ fingers/ ankle/ shoulder/ back/ wrist… hurts.
- ¿Es un dolor constante o viene y se va? – Is it constant pain or does it come and go?
- ¿Que tipo de síntomas tiene? – What kind of symptoms do you have?
- Tengo una herida. – I have a wound.
- Estoy enfermo/a. – I feel sick.
- Tengo mareos. – I feel dizzy.
- No me siento bien. – I'm not feeling well/I'm feeling sick.
- Me siento mal. – I don't feel well.
- Me siento débil. – I feel weak.
- ¿Tiene fiebre? – Do you have fever?
- Tengo un poco de fiebre. – I have a slight fever.
- Tengo fiebre alta. – I have a high fever.
- La fiebre me subió muy rápido. – The fever rose very quickly.
- Tengo fiebre desde ayer. – I have a fever since yesterday.
- Tengo - I have…
- El tiene - he has…
- Ella tiene - she has…

STUDY GLOSSARY

<u>Anatomical Terminology</u>

Abdominal cavity- the part of the body between the bottom of the ribs and the top of the thighs, containing most of the digestive and urinary systems along with some reproductive organs

ABO blood groups- The system by which human blood is classified, based on proteins occurring on red blood cells; the four classification groups are A, AB, B, and O

Abortion- termination of a pregnancy; can occur because of natural causes (called a miscarriage) or be a medical intervention

Abscess- an accumulation of pus in a body tissue, usually caused by a bacterial infection ACE inhibitor- a drug typically used to treat high blood pressure (Angiotensin-Converting Enzyme inhibitor)

Absceso- Abscess

Accident- accidente

Achilles tendon- the tendon at the back of the lower leg that connects the calf muscle to the heel bone

Acid-base balance- the mechanisms that the body uses to keep its fluids close to neutral (neither basic nor acidic) so that the body can function properly

Acidosis- a condition marked by abnormally high acid levels in the blood, associated with some forms of diabetes, lung disease, and severe kidney disease

Acid reflux- a disorder in which acid in the stomach comes up into the esophagus, because the valve separating the stomach and esophagus does not function properly

Acne- a skin condition characterized by inflamed, pus-filled areas that occur on the skin's surface, most commonly occurring during adolescence

Acquired- a word describing any condition that is not present at birth, but develops some time during life

Acquired immunodeficiency syndrome- infection by the human immunodeficiency virus (HIV), which causes a weakening of the immune system

Acute- describes a condition or illness that begins suddenly and is usually short-lasting

Acute respiratory disease- an urgent condition in which oxygen levels in the blood are lower than normal and breathing is difficult

Adaptogen- An herb that helps the body resist or adapt to physical, biological, or chemical stressors. By definition, an adaptogen is non-toxic and produces minimal or no side effects (Winston & Maimes, 2007).

Addiction- dependence on a substance (such as alcohol or other drugs) or an activity, to the point that stopping is very difficult and causes severe physical and mental reactions

Adenitis- infection and inflammation of a gland, especially a lymph node

Adipose tissue- another term for fatty tissue; it stores energy, insulates, and cushions the body

Adjuvant- Aids the action of other ingredients of a formula, e.g., encouraging assimilation, balancing energetic or other qualities, or guiding the direction of actions.

Adjuvant therapy- the use of drugs or radiation therapy in the treatment of cancer along with surgery

Adrenal failure- a condition in which the adrenal glands do not produce enough of the hormones that control important functions such as blood pressure

Adrenal glands- two small glands located on top of the kidneys that secrete several important hormones into the blood

Adverse reaction- an unintended and unwanted side effect of some sort of treatment, usually drug therapy

Aerobic exercise- physical activity during which the heart and lungs must work harder to meet the body's increased oxygen demand

Affective disorder- a mental disorder involving abnormal moods and emotions; affective disorders include manic-depressive disorder

Afterbirth- the placenta and membranes that are eliminated from the woman's uterus following the birth of a child

Afterpains- normal contractions of the uterus after childbirth that usually occur for the first few days after delivery

AIDS- see Acquired immunodeficiency syndrome
AIDS-related complex- symptoms including weight loss, fever, and enlarged lymph nodes experienced by people who are infected with HIV but do not yet have AIDS

Air embolism- the blockage of an artery by air bubbles, which may have entered during surgery or after an injury

Airway obstruction- blockage of the passage of air through the windpipe to the lungs

Airways- the passageways that air moves through while traveling in and out of the lungs during breathing

Albinism- a condition in which people are born with insufficient amounts of the pigment melanin, which is responsible for hair, skin, and eye color

Albumin- Albumin is a protein made by your liver. Albumin enters your bloodstream and helps keep fluid from leaking out of your blood vessels into other tissues. It is also carries hormones, vitamins, and enzymes throughout your body.

Alcoholic cardiomyopathy- heart damage and failure caused by intake of too much alcohol

Alimentary canal- another term for the digestive tract

Alkalosis- dangerously decreased acidity of the blood, which can be caused by high altitudes, hyperventilation, and excessive vomiting

Alkylating agents- substances used in cancer treatment that interfere with the division of cells

Allopathy- May be referred to as conventional, modern, or Western medicine. It has also been described as "A system of medical practice that aims to combat disease by use of remedies (as drugs or surgery) producing effects different from or incompatible with those produced by the disease being treated" (MerriamWebster, 2017).

Allergen- a substance that causes an allergic reaction

Allergic rhinitis- irritation of the nasal passages and the whites of the eyes, causing sneezing, runny nose, and sore eyes

Allergy- a negative reaction to a substance that in most people causes no reaction Alopecia- baldness or loss of hair, mainly on the head, either in defined patches or completely; the cause is unknown ALS- see Amyotrophic lateral sclerosis

Alterative- Describes herbs that help the body eliminate metabolic wastes and assimilate nutrients, therefore restoring normal function and vitality.

Altitude sickness- headaches, dizziness, and nausea usually experienced at heights above 8,000 ft because of reduced oxygen in the air

Alzheimer disease- a condition that occurs late in life and worsens with time in which brain cells degenerate; it is accompanied by memory loss, physical decline, and confusion

Amenorrhea- absence of menstrual periods, occurring either after or before menstruation has begun

Aminotransferase- enzymes that catalyze a transamination reaction between an amino acid and an α-keto acid. They are important in the synthesis of amino acids, which form proteins.

Amniocentesis- a procedure in which a small amount of amniotic fluid is removed from the mother's womb in order to detect abnormalities of the fetus

Amniotic fluid- clear fluid that surrounds a fetus during pregnancy and cushions and protects it

Amyotrophic lateral sclerosis- the most common of a group of disorders known as motor neuron diseases, in which the nerves in the brain that control the movement of muscles degenerate and muscle function is gradually lost; commonly called Lou Gehrig's disease

Anabolic steroid- a drug similar to the male hormone

testosterone that builds muscles and strengthens bones, but has adverse side effects

Anal fissure- a long, open sore on the skin of the anus

Anal fistula- an abnormal tubelike passage connecting the anus to the surface of the

surrounding skin

Analgesic- a drug that relieves pain, such as aspirin or acetaminophen

Anal sphincter- a ring of muscle fibers at the opening of the rectum, controlling the opening and closing of the anus

Anaphylactic shock- a life-threatening allergic reaction resulting in difficulty breathing and low blood pressure

Anatomy- the structure of bodies; commonly refers to the study of body structure Androgen- a hormone (such as testosterone) that causes development of male characteristics and sex organs

Anemia- a condition in which the blood does not contain enough hemoglobin, the compound that carries oxygen from the lungs to other parts of the body

Anencephaly- a fatal birth defect in which the brain and spinal cord have failed to develop, resulting in the absence of a portion of the skull and brain
Anesthesia- a loss of sensation in a certain part of the body or throughout the body

Anesthetic- a substance that temporarily causes a person to be unable to feel pain, either in a certain area or over the entire body

Aneurysm- an abnormal swelling of the wall of an artery, caused by a weakening in the vessel wall

Angina pectoris- pain experienced in the chest, arms, or jaw because of a lack of oxygen to the heart muscle

Angioma- a tumor made of blood vessels or lymph vessels that is not cancerous Angioplasty- the use of surgery to make a damaged blood vessel function properly again; may involve widening or reconstructing the blood vessel

Ankle- tobillo

Anodyne- Lessens pain by reducing nervous system response or perception to it.

Anorexia nervosa- a dangerous eating disorder mainly affecting young girls in which the sufferer has an intense fear of looking fat, avoids food, and loses weight excessively

Antacid- a drug that neutralizes stomach acids; used to treat indigestion, heartburn, and acid reflux

Antibiotic resistance- the development by bacteria of the ability to live in the presence of a certain antibiotic, making treatment difficult

Antibiotics- bacteria-killing substances that are used to fight infection

Antibody- a protein made by white blood cells that reacts with a specific foreign protein as part of the immune response

Anticatarrhal- Dissolves, eliminates, or impedes the formation of mucus.

Anticoagulants- drugs used to stop abnormal blood clotting, such as to prevent stroke Antiemetics- drugs used to treat nausea and vomiting

Antihistamine- a drug that relieves an allergic reaction by stopping the effects of histamine, the substance responsible for the negative symptoms associated with the reaction

Antihypertensives- drugs used to relieve the symptoms and prevent the damage that can occur from high blood pressure

Antioxidants- substances that protect against cell damage by guarding the cell from oxygen free radicals

Antipsychotics- drugs used to treat severe mental disorders

Antiseptics- chemicals applied to the skin that prevent infection by killing bacteria and other harmful organisms

Anus- the opening through which feces are passed from the body

Aorta- the main artery in the body, carrying oxygenated blood from the heart to other arteries in the body

Aortic stenosis- narrowing of the opening of the aortic valve in the heart, which increases resistance to blood flow from the left ventricle to the aorta; commonly a birth defect or caused by scarring and calcium accumulation in the valve from rheumatic fever

Aperient- Encourages the appetite or digestion, typically preparing the digestive environment. Sometimes used to describe herbs that gently promote elimination, as in a mild laxative.

Apgar score- a system for evaluating the health of a newborn baby; rated on a scale of 0- 10

Aplasia- the complete or partial failure of any organ or tissue to grow

Aplastic anemia- a severely reduced number of red blood cells, white blood cells, and platelets

Apnea- a possibly life-threatening condition in which breathing stops, for either a short or long period of time

Appendectomy- surgical removal of the appendix to treat appendicitis Appendicitis- inflammation of the appendix

Appendix- a short, tubelike structure that branches off the large intestine; does not have any known function

Appendix- apéndice

Appetite loss- pérdida de apetito

ARC- see AIDS-related complex
Arteriosclerosis- a disorder causing thickening and hardening of artery walls

Arm- brazo

Aromatherapy- A botanical approach that uses essential oils extracted from medicinal plants or other aromatic means of delivery. May be used topically, inhaled, or consumed orally (in some cases) to elicit physiological effects, often emotional, by olfactory stimulation.

Arrhythmia- arritmia

Arteritis- inflammation of the walls of an artery that causes the passageway to become narrower; can lead to tissue damage because oxygen is not properly supplied

Artery- a large blood vessel that carries blood from the heart to tissues and organs in the body

Arthritis- a disease of the joints characterized by inflammation, pain, stiffness, and redness

Arthritis- artritis

Arthroscopy- a procedure used to examine the inside of a joint using a viewing tube (an endoscope)

Artificial insemination- injection of semen into the cervix

Artificial respiration/ventilation- the forcing of air (either by mouth-to-mouth or mouth- to-nose means) into the lungs of a person who has stopped breathing

Ascites- excess fluid in the abdominal cavity, which leads to swelling Ascorbic acid- the chemical term for vitamin C

Aspermia- the failure either to produce or to ejaculate sperm

Asphyxia- the medical term for suffocation; can be caused by choking on an object, by lack of oxygen in the air, or by chemicals such as carbon monoxide, which reduce the amount of oxygen in the blood

Asthma- a disorder characterized by inflamed airways and difficulty breathing Astigmatism- a disorder in which the front surface of the eye (the cornea) is not correctly spherical, resulting in blurry vision

Astringent- Causes tissue to constrict and tighten, becoming less permeable.

Atherectomy- a procedure performed to remove plaque that is blocking an artery

Atheroma- fatty deposits on the inner walls of blood vessels, which can cause narrowing and decrease blood flow

Atherosclerosis- narrowing of the lining of the arteries due to the accumulation of fat and other materials; leads to coronary heart disease, stroke, and other disorders

Athlete's foot- an infection between the toes caused by a fungus, which leads to sore, cracked, and peeling skin

Atresia- a birth defect in which a normal body opening or canal is absent; usually requires surgical repair soon after birth

Atria- the two upper chambers of the heart; the singular form is atrium

Atrial fibrillation- an irregular heartbeat in which the upper chambers of the heart (the atria) beat inconsistently and rapidly

Atrial flutter- an irregular heartbeat in which the upper chambers of the heart (the atria) beat rapidly but consistently

Atrial septal defect- a hole located in the wall between the two upper chambers of the heart

Atrioventricular node- a node located between the atria and ventricles that regulates electrical impulse conduction between the chambers

Atrophy- the shrinkage or near disappearance of a tissue or organ

Attention-deficit disorder- a disorder mainly present in children and adolescents, characterized by learning and behavior problems, inability to pay attention, and sometimes hyperactivity

Audiogram- a graph showing a person's hearing ability, determined from a set of tests examining hearing acuity of different sound frequencies

Aura- a "warning" signal that comes before a migraine headache or an epileptic seizure, which might include emotions or sensations of movement or discomfort

Auscultation- the act of listening to sounds within the body, such as the heartbeat, with a stethoscope

Autism- a mental disorder characterized by an inability to relate to other people and extreme withdrawal

Autoimmune disease- a disorder in which the body's immune system attacks itself

Autonomic nervous system- the part of the nervous system that controls automatic body functions, such as heart rate, sweating, pupil dilation, and digestion; divided into the sympathetic nervous system and the parasympathetic nervous system

Autopsy- the examination of a body following death, possibly to determine the cause of death or for research

Autosomal dominant- a term describing a gene on any chromosome other than the sex chromosomes that produces its effect whenever it is present; can also describe the effect of the gene itself

Autosomal recessive- a term used to describe a gene on any chromosome other than the sex chromosomes that produces its effect only when two copies of it are present; can also describe the effect of the gene itself

Axilla- medical term for the armpit

Ayurveda- Translates to "science of life" and is the subset of teachings referring to an ancient Indian medical system including food, herbs, exercise, and lifestyle recommendations to support vibrant health. This system has a recognizable characteristic of using approaches that are personalized according to a person's constitution (prakriti) and the three mind/body types (doshas).

B

Bacillus- any bacteria that is rod-shaped; responsible for diphtheria, dysentery, tetanus, and tuberculosis, as well as other diseases

Back- espalda

Bacteremia- a condition in which bacteria are present in the bloodstream; may occur after minor surgery or infection and may be dangerous for people with a weakened immune system or abnormal heart valves

Bacterial infection- infección bacteriana

Bacteriostatic- term used to describe a substance that stops the growth of bacteria (such as an antibiotic)

Bacterium- a tiny, single-celled microorganism, commonly known as a germ; some bacteria, called pathogens, cause disease

Bacteriuria- bacteria in the urine; large amounts can indicate bladder, urethra, or kidney infection

Ball-and-socket joint- a joint consisting of a ball-shaped bone that fits into a cup-shaped bone, making the joint free to rotate; examples include the hip and shoulder

Balloon angioplasty- a technique that uses a balloon catheter to open arteries clogged with fatty deposits

Balloon catheter- a hollow tube with a small, inflatable balloon at the tip; used to open a narrowed artery or organ that has become blocked

Bang your head- golpearse la cabeza

Barbiturates- a group of sedatives that reduce activity in the brain; are habit-forming and are possibly fatal when taken with alcohol

Barium enema- a technique in which barium is placed into the large intestine and rectum and then X-rays are taken to check for possible disorders of these organs

Barrier method of contraception- a birth-control technique using a condom, diaphragm, or another similar device to block the path of sperm to an egg

Bartholin's glands- two pea-sized glands that, when sexually aroused, release a fluid that lubricates the vagina

Basal cell carcinoma- a type of skin cancer that is caused by exposure to large amounts of sunlight; commonly found on the neck, face, and arms

Basal metabolic rate- the lowest rate at which a person can possibly use energy and remain alive; at this rate, only absolutely necessary functions such as breathing are maintained

B cell- a white blood cell that makes antibodies to fight infections caused by foreign proteins

BCG vaccine- a vaccine used to protect against tuberculosis

Becker's muscular dystrophy- a hereditary disease in which the muscles weaken and waste away; similar to Duchenne muscular dystrophy but starts later in life and advances more slowly

Bell's palsy- another name for facial palsy, the usually one-sided, temporary numbing of the facial muscles, caused by an inflamed nerve

Bends- see Decompression sickness
Benign tumor- a tumor that is not cancerous, which means it does not spread through the body, but may grow and become dangerous

Beta blocker- a type of drug used to treat high blood pressure and heart disorders by reducing the strength and rate of the pumping by the heart

Beta carotene- a pigment found in orange vegetables and fruits, which the body converts to vitamin A; possibly protects against cancer

Bifocal- a lens that corrects both near and distant vision by having two parts with different focusing strengths

Bilateral- a term describing a condition that affects both sides of the body or two paired organs, such as bilateral deafness (deafness in both ears)

Bile- a yellow-green liquid produced in the liver whose function is to remove waste from the liver and break down fats as food is digested

Bile duct- a tube that carries bile from the liver to the gallbladder and then to the small intestine

Biliary atresia- a birth defect in which the bile ducts are not completely developed; often a liver transplant is necessary

Biliary colic- a severe pain in the upper right section of the abdomen, usually caused by a gallstone passing out of the bladder or through the bile ducts

Biliary tract- the system of organs and ducts through which bile is made and transported from the liver to the small intestine

Bilirubin- the orange-yellow pigment in bile, causing jaundice if it builds up in the blood and skin; the levels of bilirubin in the blood are used to diagnose liver disease

Binging and purging- behavior characteristic of the disorder bulimia in which a person overeats then rids themselves of the food before it can be absorbed by the body, either by forced vomiting or through the use of laxatives

Biochemistry- the science that studies the chemistry of living organisms, including humans

Bioequivalent- a drug that has the same effect on the body as another drug

Biofeedback- a technique used to gain control over a function that is normally automatic (such as blood pressure or pulse rate); the function is monitored and relaxation techniques are used to change it to a desired level

Bipolar disorder- an illness in which the patient goes back and forth between opposite extremes; the most notable bipolar disorder is manic-depressive disorder, which is characterized by extreme highs and lows in mood

Birth canal- the passage that includes the uterus and vagina through which the baby passes at birth

Birth control- the regulation of the number of children born, referring either to the prevention of pregnancy (by birth control pill, sterilization, etc) or the prevention of birth (by abortion, etc)

Birth defect- an abnormality that is present when a baby is born

Birthmark- any area of discolored skin that is present when a baby is born

Bisexuality- sexual interest in members of both sexes

Bitter- Encourages digestive secretions and good digestive function typically by the action on bitter taste receptors. Constituents with this action may also stimulate repair mechanisms in the gut

Bladder- an organ located in the pelvis whose function is to collect and store urine until it is expelled

Bleed / bleeding- sangrar / hemorragia

Bleeding- sangrado

Blepharitis- inflammation of the eyelids

Blind spot- a spot in the field of vision that is not sensitive to light; it is a product of the entrance of the optic nerve into the eyeball, where no light receptors are present on the retina

Blood-brain barrier- a layer of tightly bound cells that prevents certain substances carried in the bloodstream from entering the brain

Blood clot- a semisolid mass of blood that forms to help seal and prevent bleeding from a damaged vessel

Blood poisoning- see Septicemia

Blood pressure- the tension in the main arteries that is created by the beating of the heart

and the resistance to flow and elasticity of the blood vessels

Blood transfusion- the transfer of blood or any of its parts to a person who has lost blood due to an injury, disease, or operation

Blood type- a category used to describe a person's blood according to the kinds of proteins present on the surface of the red blood cells

B lymphocyte- a type of white blood cell that makes antibodies and is an important part of the immune response

Boil- an inflamed, raised area of skin that is pus-filled; usually an infected hair follicle Bone marrow- the fatty yellow or red tissue inside bones that is responsible for producing blood cells

Bone marrow transplant- a surgical procedure in which defective or cancerous bone marrow is replaced with healthy marrow, either from the patient or a donor

Bone spur- an abnormal growth of bone out of another bone, often located on the heel and usually painful

Booster- an additional dose of a vaccine taken after the first dose to maintain or renew the first one

Botulism- poisoning from poorly preserved food contaminated with a dangerous bacterial toxin that results in paralysis

Bowel- see Intestine

Bradycardia- a slow heart rate, usually below 60 beats per minute in adults

Brain- cerebro

Brain damage- permanent death or damage of brain cells resulting in decreased mental ability

Brain death- the condition in which the brain stops functioning while the heart continues to beat

Break a bone- romperse un hueso

breathing difficulty / shortness of breath- dificultad respiratoria

Breech birth- childbirth in which the baby is turned around in the uterus and emerges head-last instead of head-first

Bronchiolitis- an infection caused by a virus in the bronchioles (the smallest airways in the lungs), mainly affecting young children

Bronchitis- inflammation of the bronchial tubes, which connect the trachea to the lungs

Bronchoconstrictor- a substance that causes the lung airways to tighten up and become more narrow

Bronchodilator- a drug that widens the airways in the lungs to improve breathing; works by relieving muscle contraction or buildup of mucus

Bronchospasm- the temporary narrowing of the airways in the lungs, either as a result of muscle contraction or inflammation; may be caused by asthma, infection, lung disease, or an allergic reaction

Bruise- see Contusion

Bruise- moretón

Bruxism- an unaware clenching or grinding of the teeth, usually during sleep Bubonic plague- a form of plague in which lymph nodes in the groin and armpit swell

BUN (Blood Urea Nitrogen)- Produced by the liver... Urea nitrogen is a waste product that your kidneys remove from your blood. Higher than normal BUN levels may be a sign that your kidneys aren't working well.

Bulimia- a disorder in which a person eats large amounts of food then forces vomiting or uses laxatives to prevent weight gain (called binging and purging)

Bunion- a hard, fluid-filled pad along the inside joint of the big toe; may be caused by wearing high-heeled shoes or a genetically weak joint

Burkitt's lymphoma- a cancer of lymph tissue that most frequently occurs in the abdomen, the ovaries, and the bones of the face; it is associated with malaria

Burn- quemaduras

Bursa- a fluid-filled sac that cushions and reduces friction in certain parts of the body Bursitis- inflammation of a bursa due to excessive pressure or friction, or from injury

Butterfly bandage- a butterfly-shaped bandage that can help close a minor cut for proper healing

Bypass- a surgical technique in which the flow of blood or another body fluid is redirected around a blockage

C

C reactive protein- a protein made by the liver. The level of **CRP** increases when there's inflammation in the body.

Calcification- the depositing of calcium salts in the body, which occurs normally in teeth and bones but abnormally in injured muscles and narrowed arteries

Calcitonin- a hormone made in the thyroid gland that controls calcium levels in the blood by slowing the loss of calcium from bones; used to treat hypercalcemia (excess calcium in the blood)

Calcium- a plentiful mineral in the body and the basic component of teeth and bones; essential for cell function, muscle contraction, transmission of nerve impulses, and blood clotting

Calcium channel blocker- a drug used to treat chest pain, high blood pressure, and irregular heartbeat by preventing the movement of calcium into the muscle

Callus- a thickened area of skin due to consistent pressure or friction, or the area around a bone break where new bone is formed

Calorie- a unit that is used to measure the energy content in food
Canal- a tunnel-like passage

Cancer- a group of diseases in which cells grow unrestrained in an organ or tissue in the body; can spread to tissues around it and destroy them or be transported through blood or lymph pathways to other parts of the body

Cancer- cáncer

Cancer staging- a method to determine how much a cancer has developed

Candidiasis- a yeast infection caused by the fungus Candida albicans; occurs most often in the vagina, but also in the mouth, on moist skin, or on the penis

Canker sore- small, painful sore that usually occurs on the inside of the lip or cheek, or sometimes under the tongue; caused by bacteria, irritation of the area, stress, or allergies

Capillary- a tiny blood vessel that connects the smallest arteries to the smallest veins and allows exchange of oxygen and other materials between blood cells and body tissue cells

Car accident- accidente de auto

Carbohydrate- a substance, mainly sugar and starch, that is a main source of energy for the body and is found in sources such as cereals, breads, pastas, grains, and vegetables

Carbon dioxide- a colorless, odorless gas present in small amounts in the atmosphere and formed during respiration

Carcinogen- anything that can cause cancer
Carcinoma- a cancer that occurs on the surface or lining of an organ

Cardiac arrest- the sudden cessation of the heart's pumping action, possibly due to a heart attack, respiratory arrest, electrical shock, extreme cold, blood loss, drug overdose, or a severe allergic reaction

Cardiogenic shock- a severely dangerous condition involving decreased blood output from the heart, usually as a result of a heart attack

Cardiomegaly- a condition marked by enlargement of the heart, either because of a thickened heart muscle or an enlarged heart chamber; usually a result of the heart having to work harder than normal, as occurs with high blood pressure

Cardiomyopathy- a disease of the heart muscle that results in decreased output and reduced blood flow

Cardiopulmonary resuscitation- the administration of heart compression and artificial respiration to restore circulation and breathing

Cardiovascular system- the heart and blood vessels that are responsible for circulating blood throughout the body

Carditis- inflammation of the heart

Carminative- Spice or herb with an aromatic quality that promotes digestion and soothes the gastrointestinal tract, leading to less cramping, bloating, and gas.

Carotene- an orange pigment present in colored plants such as carrots that is converted by the body to the essential nutrient vitamin A

Carotid arteries- four main arteries that carry blood to the head and neck

Carpal bones- eight bones that together make the wrist

Carpal tunnel syndrome- a condition in which pressure on the median nerve in the wrist causes soreness, tingling, and numbness in the thumb and index and middle fingers

Cartilage- a connective tissue (softer than bone) that is part of the skeletal system, including the joints

Cast- a hard plaster or fiberglass shell that molds to a body part such as an arm and holds it in place for proper healing

Cataract- a disorder in which the lens of the eye becomes less transparent and in some cases a milky white, making vision less clear

Catheter- a hollow, flexible tube inserted into the body to put in or take out fluid, or to open up or close blood vessels

Catheterization- a technique in which a hollow, flexible tube is used to drain body fluids (such as urine), to introduce fluids into the body, or to examine or widen a narrowed vein or artery

CAT scanning- see Computed tomography scanning

Cat-scratch fever- an illness transmitted to humans through a cat's bite or scratch, which is thought to be caused by an unidentified bacteria; characterized by a swollen lymph node or blister near the bite or scratch, fever, rash, and headache; most commonly occurring in children

Cauliflower ear- a deformed ear caused by repeated injury

Cauterization- the use of heat, an electric current, or a chemical to destroy tissue or stop bleeding

CBC test- A complete blood count, also known as a full blood count, is a set of medical laboratory tests that provide information about the cells in a person's blood. The CBC indicates the counts of white blood cells, red blood cells and platelets, the concentration of hemoglobin, and the hematocrit.

Cecum- the beginning of the large intestine, which is connected to the appendix at its lower end

Cell- the tiny structures that make up all the tissues of the body and carry out all of its functions

Cellulitis- a skin infection caused by bacteria (usually streptococci); can lead to tissue damage and blood poisoning if untreated; characterized by fever, chills, heat, tenderness, and redness

Central nervous system- the brain and spinal cord

Cerebellum- a region of the brain located at the back; responsible for coordination of movement and maintaining balance

Cerebral palsy- a group of disorders of movement and posture resulting from damage to the brain early in a child's development; causes muscle weakness, difficulty coordinating voluntary movements, and sometimes complete loss of motion

Cerebrospinal fluid- a clear, watery fluid circulating in and around the brain and spinal column, which contains glucose, proteins, and salts for nutrition

Cerebrovascular disease- a disease affecting any artery supplying blood to the brain; may cause blockage or rupture of a blood vessel, leading to a stroke

Cerebrum- the largest part of the brain and the site of most of its activity, including sensory and motor functions

Cervical cap- a small rubber cup that is placed tightly over the cervix to prevent pregnancy

Cervical dysplasia- changes that occur in the cells on the surface of the cervix that usually precede the stages of cancer

Cervical incompetence- a weakness of the neck of the uterus, which can lead to spontaneous abortion due to an inability to support the weight of the fetus

Cervical smear- a procedure in which cells are scraped off of the cervix and examined to detect changes that might precede the stages of cancer; also called a Pap smear

Cervicitis- inflammation of the cervix

Cervix- a small, round organ making up the neck of the uterus and separating it from the vagina

Cesarean section- an operation performed to remove a fetus by cutting into the uterus, usually through the abdominal wall

Chancre- a painless sore that has a thick, rubbery base and a defined edge; usually occurs on the genitals after the contraction of the sexually transmitted disease syphilis

Chem 7 test- looks at seven different substances in the blood, Blood urea nitrogen (BUN), Carbon dioxide, Creatinine, Glucose, Serum chloride, Serum potassium, Serum sodium

Chemotherapy- the treatment of infections or cancer with drugs that act on disease- producing organisms or cancerous tissue; may also affect normal cells

Chest- pecho

Chickenpox- a contagious disease that causes a rash and a fever; most commonly occurs during childhood

Chlamydia- microorganisms that cause several human infections and can be transmitted sexually

Cholagogue- Stimulates the flow of bile, supporting digestive processes. Often bitter in nature.

Cholecystectomy- the surgical removal of the gallbladder

Cholera- a bacterial infection of the small intestine that causes severe watery diarrhea, dehydration, and possibly death

Cholesterol- a substance in body cells that plays a role in the production of hormones and bile salts and in the transport of fats in the bloodstream

Chondritis- inflammation of cartilage

Chondroma- a noncancerous tumor that occurs in cartilage

Chondromalacia patellae- painful damage to the cartilage behind the kneecap

Chondrosarcoma- a cancerous cartilage tumor that develops inside of bone or on its surface

Chorionic villus sampling- a method of diagnosing fetal defects in which a small amount of tissue is taken from the placenta and analyzed for abnormalities

Choroiditis- inflammation of the blood vessels behind the retina that line the back of the eye

Chromosome analysis- examination of a person's chromosomes either to determine if that person has an abnormality or to investigate one

Chronic- describes a disorder that continues for a long period of time

Chronic obstructive lung disease- a combination of the lung diseases emphysema and bronchitis, characterized by blockage of airflow in and out of the lungs

Cilia- tiny, hairlike structures on the outside of some cells, providing mobility

Circumcision- the surgical removal of the foreskin of the penis

Cirrhosis of the liver- gradual loss of liver function due to cell damage and internal scarring

Claudication- a cramping pain in one or both legs while walking, which can cause limping

Claustrophobia- fear of being confined in an enclosed or crowded space

Clavicle- the medical term for the collarbone

Cleft lip- a birth defect in which the upper lip is split vertically, extending into one or both nostrils

Cleft palate- a birth defect in which the roof of the mouth is split, extending from behind the teeth to the nasal cavity; often occurs with other birth defects such as cleft lip and partial deafness

Clinical trial- carefully monitored and planned testing of a new drug or treatment

Clitoris- a small female organ located near the opening of the vagina that swells when sexually aroused

Clone- an exact copy of a gene, cell, or organism

Closed fracture- a bone break that does not break the skin

Clotting factor- a substance in the blood that is needed for blood to harden and stop a wound from bleeding

Clubfoot- a genetic disorder in which the foot is twisted and misshapen

Cluster headache- severe pain that occurs suddenly and affects one side of the head, including the face and neck

CNS- see Central nervous system

Coagulation- a process that plays a large role in the hardening and thickening of blood to form a clot

Cocarcinogen- a substance that does not cause cancer by itself, but increases the effect of a substance that does cause cancer

Coccyx- four fused bones that form a triangular shape at the base of the spine (also known as the tailbone)

Cochlea- a coiled organ in the inner ear that plays a large role in hearing by picking up sound vibrations and transmitting them as electrical signals

Coitus- sexual intercourse

Cognitive Behavioral Therapy (CBT)- terapia cognitivo conductual (TCC)

Cold sore- a small blister anywhere around the mouth that is caused by the herpes simplex virus

Colectomy- the complete or partial surgical removal of the large intestine (the colon), usually as treatment of a cancerous tumor or a narrowing and blockage of the intestine

Colic- waves of pain in the abdomen that increase in strength, disappear, and return; usually caused by a stone blocking a bile or urine passageway or an intestinal infection

Colitis- inflammation of the large intestine (the colon), which usually leads to abdominal pain, fever, and diarrhea with blood and mucus

Collapsed lung- a condition in which all or part of a lung cannot expand and fill with air

Colon- the main part of the large intestine, between the cecum and the rectum

Colon- colon

Colonoscopy- investigation of the inside of the colon using a long, flexible fiberoptic tube

Color blindness- any vision disorder in which the person sees colors abnormally, has trouble distinguishing between them, or cannot see them at all

Colostomy- a surgical procedure in which some part of the colon is cut and moved to the surface of the abdomen so that feces can be passed into a bag worn outside of the body

Coma- a condition in which the area of the brain involved in maintaining consciousness is somehow affected, resulting in a state of unconsciousness in which the patient does not respond to stimulation

Comminuted fracture- a crushed or shattered bone

Common cold- an infection caused by a virus, which results in an inflamed lining of the nose and throat; characterized by a stuffy and runny nose and, sometimes, a sore throat

Communicable disease- a disease that can be passed from one individual to another

Compound fracture- a bone break that breaks the skin

Compression fracture- a break in a short bone in which its soft tissue is crushed

Computed tomography scanning- a technique for producing cross-sectional images of the body in which X-rays are passed through the body at different angles and analyzed by a computer; also called CT scanning or CAT scanning

Concussion- disturbance of electrical activity in the brain due to a blow to the head or neck, causing temporary loss of consciousness

Congenital- present or existing at the time of birth

Congestive heart failure- inability of the heart to efficiently pump blood through the body, causing buildup of blood in the veins and of other body fluids in tissue

Conjunctiva- the clear membrane covering the white of the eye and the inside of the eyelid that produces a fluid that lubricates the cornea and eyelid

Conjunctivitis- inflammation of the conjunctiva; commonly called pinkeye

Connective tissue- strong tissue that connects and supports body structures

Constipation- difficult or infrequent bowel movements of hard, dry feces

Constipation- estreñimiento

Contraindication- an aspect of a patient's condition that makes the use of a certain drug or therapy an unwise or dangerous decision

Contusion- damage to the skin and underlying tissue as a result of a blunt injury; a bruise

Corn- a thickened callus on the foot that is caused by an improperly fitting shoe

Cornea- the clear, dome-shaped front portion of the eye's outer covering

Coronary- describes structures that encircle another structure (such as the coronary arteries, which circle the heart); commonly used to refer to a coronary thrombosis or a heart attack

Coronary arteries- the arteries that branch off from the aorta and supply oxygen-rich blood to the heart muscle

Coronary artery bypass surgery- an operation in which a piece of vein or artery is used to bypass a blockage in a coronary artery; performed to prevent myocardial infarction and relieve angina pectoris

Coronary heart disease- disorders that restrict the blood supply to the heart, including atherosclerosis

Coronary thrombosis- the blockage of a coronary artery by a blood clot Corpuscle- a tiny, rounded structure in the body, such as a red or white blood cell

Corticosteroids- synthetic drugs that are used to replace natural hormones or to suppress the immune system and help prevent inflammation

Cough- tos

CPR- see Cardiopulmonary resuscitation
Creatinine- a waste product that is filtered from the blood by the kidneys and expelled in urine

Creatinine- Creatinine is a breakdown product of creatine phosphate from muscle and protein metabolism. It is released at a constant rate by the body. Healthy kidneys filter creatinine out of the blood. Creatinine exits your body as a waste product in urine.

Croup- a usually mild and temporary condition common in children under the age of 4 in which the walls of the airways become inflamed and narrow, resulting in wheezing and coughing

Cruciate ligaments- two ligaments in the knee that cross each other and help stabilize the knee joint

CT scanning- a procedure that uses X-rays and computers to create cross-sectional images of the body to diagnose and monitor disease

Culture- the artificial growth of cells, tissue, or microorganisms such as bacteria in a laboratory

Curative therapy- terapia curativa

Curettage- the use of a sharp, spoonlike instrument (a curet) to scrape away tissue that is abnormal or to obtain a sample that can be analyzed

To cut / cut- cortarse / corte

CVS- see Chorionic villus sampling

Cyanosis- a bluish discoloration of the skin, caused by low levels of oxygen in the blood

Cyst- a lump filled with either fluid or soft material, occurring in any organ or tissue; may occur for a number of reasons but is usually harmless unless its presence disrupts organ or tissue function

Cystectomy- surgical removal of the bladder; the bladder is often replaced with a short length of small intestine

Cystic fibrosis- an inherited disorder in which the lungs are prone to infection, and fats and other nutrients cannot be absorbed into the body

Cystoscopy- examination of the urethra and bladder using a long, thin, fiberoptic tube

Cystostomy- the surgical placement of a drainage opening in the bladder

Cytokines - a broad and loose category of small proteins (~5–25 kDa) important in cell signaling. Cytokines have been classed as lymphokines, interleukins, and chemokines, based on their presumed cell of secretion, function, or target of action.

D

D and C- see Dilatation and Curettage

Debilitation / weakness- debilitamiento / debilidad

Debridement- surgical removal of dead, damaged, or infected tissue, or some foreign material from a wound or burn

Decompression sickness- the formation of gas bubbles in the body's tissues as a result of a scuba diver ascending too quickly from depth; commonly called the bends

Deep-vein thrombosis- the formation of a blood clot inside of a deep-lying vein, usually in the legs

Defecation- the passing of feces out of the body through the anus; a bowel movement

Defibrillation- a short electric shock to the chest to normalize an irregular heartbeat

Degenerative arthritis- the breakdown of the cartilage lining the bones in joints, usually weight-bearing joints (such as the knee); causes stiffness and pain (also called osteoarthritis)

Dehydration- excessive, dangerous loss of water from the body

Dehydration- deshidratación

Demulcent- Rich in mucilage, a slippery substance that soothes, cools, and protects irritated or inflamed internal tissue that is raw, hot, irritated, inflamed, or overexcited

Dementia- a gradual decline in mental ability usually caused by a brain disease, such as Alzheimer disease

Depilatory- a chemical hair remover

Depot injection- injection of a drug into a muscle; the drug is designed to absorb slowly into the body

Depression- feelings of hopelessness, sadness, and a general disinterest in life, which for the most part have no cause and may be the result of a psychiatric illness

Depression- depresión

Dermabrasion- removal of the surface layer of skin with a sanding wheel to treat scarring or to remove tattoos

Dermatitis- inflammation of the skin Dermis- the inner skin layer

Desensitization- the process of making a person less allergic to a substance by injecting gradually increasing amounts of the substance; sometimes done to prevent anaphylactic shock

Detoxification- treatment given either to fight a person's dependence on alcohol or other drugs or to rid the body of a poisonous substance and its effects

Dextrocardia- a rare genetic condition in which the heart is located on the right side of the body, instead of the left

Dextrose- another name for the sugar glucose

Diabetes- diabetes

Diabetes insipidus- a rare condition characterized by increased urine production

Diabetes mellitus- a common form of diabetes in which the body cannot properly store or use glucose (sugar), the body's main source of energy

Dialectical Behavioral Therapy (DBT)- terapia dialéctica conductual (TDC/DBT)

Dialysis- a procedure to treat kidney failure in which artificial means are used to filter waste, maintain acid-base balance, and remove excess fluid from the body

Diaper rash- a common condition in babies in which the skin in the diaper area becomes irritated and red, usually because of exposure to urine, feces, or heat

Diaphoretic- Promotes sweating and elimination of waste from the pores of the skin. In the case of a fever, promotes natural progression of changes in temperature regulation.

Diaphragm- the large, dome-shaped muscle separating the abdomen and chest that contracts and relaxes to make breathing possible; also, a thin, rubber dome that is used as a method of female contraception

Diarrhea- diarrea

Diastolic pressure- the blood pressure measured when the heart is at rest between beats

Diathermy- the use of high-frequency currents, microwaves, or ultrasound to produce heat in the body to increase blood flow, relieve pain, or destroy diseased tissue

Diet- dieta

Dilatation and Curettage- a procedure in which the vagina and cervix are widened and the lining of the uterus is scraped away to diagnose and treat disorders of the uterus

Diphtheria- a bacterial infection that causes a fever, headache, sore throat, and possibly death; diphtheria is rare in developed countries

Disk prolapse- a disorder in which one of the disks located between the vertebrae in the spine breaks down and the pulpy interior squeezes out, causing pressure on a nerve; commonly called a "slipped" or "ruptured" disk

Dislocation- displacement of the two bones in a joint

Distention- swelling, enlargement, or stretching

Diuretic- a drug that increases the amount of water in the urine, removing excess water from the body; used in treating high blood pressure and fluid retention

Diverticulitis- inflammation of diverticula (small sacs in the intestine's inner lining); can cause fever, pain, and tenderness

Dizziness- mareo

DNA- deoxyribonucleic acid; responsible for passing genetic information in nearly all organisms

Dominant gene- a gene that always produces its effect when it is present

Dopamine- a chemical that transmits messages in the brain and plays a role in movement

Down syndrome- a genetic disorder in which a person's cells have 1 too many chromosomes, causing moderate to severe mental handicap and a characteristic appearance

Drug therapy / pharmacotherapy- farmacoterapia

Duchenne muscular dystrophy- a genetic condition in boys in which nerves degenerate and muscles get progressively weaker

Duodenal ulcer- an erosion in the inner lining of the wall of the first part of the small intestine (called the duodenum)

Duodenum- the first part of the small intestine, immediately following the stomach

Dysentery- a severe intestinal infection, causing abdominal pain and diarrhea with blood or mucus

Dyspnea- difficulty breathing

Dystrophy- any disorder in which cells become damaged or do not develop properly because they do not receive adequate nutrition

E

Eardrum- a thin, oval-shaped membrane that separates the inner ear from the outer ear and is responsible for transmitting sound waves

Ears- oídos / orejas

ECG (sometimes called an EKG)- an electrocardiogram, which is a record of the electrical impulses that trigger the heartbeat; used to diagnose heart disorders

Echocardiogram- an image of the heart that is created by high-frequency (ultrasound) sound waves

Eclampsia- a serious condition that occurs in late pregnancy, characterized by seizures in the woman

Ectopic- occurring at an abnormal position or time

Eczema- inflammation of the skin, usually causing itchiness and sometimes blisters and scaling; may be caused by allergies, but often occurs for no apparent reason

Edema- abnormal buildup of fluid in the body, which may cause visible swelling

EEG- see Electroencephalography

Elective- describes a treatment or procedure that is not urgent and can be arranged at the patient's convenience

Electrocardiogram- A printout from an electrocardiography machine used to measure and record the electrical activity of the heart.

Electrocution- descarga eléctrica

Electroencephalography- a procedure for recording the electrical impulses of brain activity

Embolism- the blockage of a blood vessel by an embolus - something previously circulating in the blood (such as a blood clot, gas bubble, tissue, bacteria, bone marrow, cholesterol, fat, etc)

Embolism- embolia

Embryo- a term used to describe a child in the womb from fertilization to 8 weeks following fertilization

Emergency room- sala de emergencias

Emetic- a substance that causes vomiting; used to treat some cases of poisoning and drug overdose

Emmenagogue- Impacts the menstrual process by stimulating and regulating menstrual flow and normalizing hormonal levels, often through their action on the liver.

Emphysema- a chronic disease in which the small air sacs in the lungs (the alveoli) become damaged; characterized by difficulty breathing

Encephalitis- inflammation of the brain, usually caused by a virus; may be very mild and barely noticeable, but is usually serious and can progress from headache and fever to hallucinations, paralysis, and sometimes coma

Endarterectomy- surgery performed to remove the lining of an artery that has been narrowed by fatty tissue buildup

Endemic- describes a disease that is always present in a certain population of people

Endocarditis- inflammation of the inner lining of the heart, usually the heart valves; typically caused by an infection

Endocardium- the inner lining of the heart

Endocrine gland- a gland that secretes hormones into the bloodstream

Endogenous- arising from inside of the body

Endometrial polyp- a growth (usually noncancerous) occurring on the lining of the uterus

Endometriosis- a condition in which fragments of the endometrium are found in other pelvic organs

Endometrium- the membrane that lines the uterus

Endophthalmitis- inflammation of the inside of the eye

Endorphin- a group of chemicals produced in the brain that reduce pain and positively affect mood

Endoscope- a lighted instrument used to view the inside of a body cavity

Endothelium- the layer of flat cells that lines the blood and lymph vessels, the heart, and other structures in the body

Endotracheal tube- a plastic tube that is fed down into the trachea through the mouth or nose to supply oxygen to a person who is not breathing properly

Enteritis- inflammation of the small intestine, usually causing diarrhea

Enterobiasis- infestation by a pinworm

Enuresis- the medical term for wetting the bed

Enzyme- a chemical, originating in a cell, that regulates reactions in the body

Epidemic- a term used to describe a disease that is rare then suddenly affects more people than usually expected

Epidermis- the outer layer of the skin

Epididymis- a long, coiled tube, exiting from the back of the testicle, in which sperm mature

Epidural anesthesia- a method of pain relief in which a painkilling drug is injected into the space surrounding the spinal cord to block sensations in the abdomen and lower body

Epilepsy- a disorder of the nervous system in which abnormal electrical activity in the brain causes seizures

Epinephrine- a hormone produced by the adrenal glands in response to stress, exercise, or fear; increases heart rate and opens airways to improve breathing; also called adrenaline

Episcleritis- a patch of inflammation on the outer layer of the white of the eye

Episiotomy- a surgical procedure in which an incision is made in the tissue between the vagina and anus to prevent tearing of this tissue during childbirth

Epithelium- the layer of cells that covers the body and lines many organs

Epstein-Barr virus- a virus that is the cause of mononucleosis and is involved in Burkitt's lymphoma

ERCP test- It is a procedure that looks at the bile and pancreatic ducts.

Erysipelas- an infection caused by streptococci bacteria; characterized by fever and rash

Erythema- redness of the skin

Erythrocyte- a red blood cell

Erythrocyte sedimentation rate- a measure of the time it takes for red blood cells to collect at the bottom of a sample of blood; an elevated rate may mean that there is inflammation somewhere in the body

Erythroplakia- red patches in the mucous membranes of the mouth, throat, or voice box (larynx) that can become cancerous; risk factors include smoking pipes and chewing tobacco

Esophageal spasm- irregular contractions of the muscles in the esophagus, which lead to difficulty swallowing

Esophageal varices- swollen veins in the lower esophagus and possibly the upper part of the stomach; can cause vomiting of blood and passing of black stool

Esophagus- a tube-shaped canal in the digestive tract, connecting the throat to the stomach

Estrogen- a group of hormones (produced mainly in the ovaries) that are necessary for female sexual development and reproductive functioning

Estrogen replacement therapy- treatment with synthetic estrogen drugs to relieve symptoms of menopause and to help protect women against osteoporosis and heart disease

Eustachian tube- the tube that connects the middle ear and the back of the nose, draining the middle ear and regulating air pressure

Euthanasia- painlessly ending the life of a patient with an incurable disease who requests to die

Excision- the surgical removal of diseased tissue

Excretion- the process by which the body rids itself of waste

Exercise stress test- the monitoring of the heart during strenuous exercise, usually on a treadmill or exercise bicycle, to evaluate how the heart responds to stress

Exercise thallium test- an imaging test performed during and after an exercise stress test to evaluate functioning of the heart muscles

Exogenous- arising from outside of the body

Expectorant- a medication used to promote the coughing up of phlegm from the respiratory tract

Extensor muscle- a muscle that causes a joint or limb to straighten

External version- external repositioning of the fetus in the womb to the correct birth position

Extracorporeal shock wave lithotripsy- a procedure performed to destroy kidney stones using external shock waves

Extract- Any of a number of related preparations intended to concentrate and preserve the active constituents of plants. Extracts include tinctures, which are a liquid extract of a plant prepared with fresh or dried plant material and a solution of alcohol and water (menstruum) often at a standard ratio of 1:5 (1 part herb by weight to 5 parts liquid by volume). A fluid extract is a concentrated tincture prepared at a 1:1 ratio.

Extradural anesthesia- injection of an anesthetic into the space outside the dura mater, the fibrous membrane that envelops the spinal cord

Eye- ojo

F

Facial palsy- inability to move the muscles of the face, usually on only one side, due to inflammation of a nerve

Failure to thrive- describes a baby who grows and gains weight slower than expected

To faint / faint- desmayarse / desmayo

To fall / fall- caerse / caída

Fallopian tube- either of two long, slender ducts connecting a woman's uterus to her ovaries, where eggs are transported from the ovaries to the uterus and sperm may fertilize an egg

Familial- a term describing a disorder or characteristic (such as male pattern baldness) that occurs within a family more often than would be expected

Fasciitis- inflammation of the layer of connective tissue that covers, separates, and supports muscles

Fatigue- fatiga

Fatty acid- any of a number of carbon-, oxygen-, and hydrogen-containing molecules that make up fats

Febrifuge- Promotes the natural process and resolution of fevers, resulting in return to normal temperature.

Febrile- a term used to describe something related to a fever, such as febrile seizures (seizures occurring in a child who has a fever)

Fecal occult blood test- a test that uses a piece of chemically sensitive paper to detect blood in a stool sample; used to screen for possible signs of cancer in the large intestine or rectum

Femoral artery- the main artery that supplies blood to the leg

Femur- the bone located between the hip and the knee; the thighbone

Fertility- the ability to produce a child

Fertility drug- a drug used to treat infertility that contains hormones or substances associated with hormones

Fertilization- the joining of an egg and a sperm, creating the first cell of a new life

Fetal alcohol syndrome- a combination of defects in a fetus as a result of the mother drinking alcohol during pregnancy

Fetal distress- physical distress experiencd by a fetus because of lack of oxygen

Fetal monitoring- the use of an instrument to record or listen to a fetus' heartbeat during pregnancy and labor

Fetal tissue transplant- an experimental procedure in which cells are taken from an aborted fetus and placed into the brain of a person with a brain disease such as Parkinson's

Fetus- the term used to refer to an unborn child from 8 weeks after fertilization to birth Fiber- a constituent of plants that cannot be digested, which helps maintain healthy functioning of the bowels

Fever- fiebre

Fiberoptics- thin, flexible instruments that transmit light and images, allowing structures inside of the body to be viewed

Fibrillation- rapid, inefficient contraction of muscle fibers of the heart caused by disruption of nerve impulses

Fibroadenoma- a noncancerous tumor commonly found in the breast

Fibrocystic breast disease- the most common cause of breast lumps

Fibroid- a noncancerous tumor of the uterus made up of smooth muscle and connective tissue

Fibroma- a noncancerous tumor of connective tissue

Fibrosis- abnormal formation of connective or scar tissue

Fifth disease- a childhood infection caused by a virus, which often starts as a rash on the cheeks and spreads

Finger- dedo (de la mano)

Fissure- a groove or slit on the body or in an organ
Fistula- an abnormal passageway from one organ to another or from an organ to the body surface

Fitness- a measure of a person's physical strength, flexibility, and endurance

Flatulence- excessive air or gas in the intestines, which is expelled through the anus

Floaters- small spots that float across the field of vision, caused by debris floating in the gel-like substance that fills the eye

Flower Essences- Developed by Dr. Bach in the 1930s, this approach infuses flowers or other parts of plants in spring water preserved with a small amount of alcohol. Resultant essences are used topically or internally to influence emotional well-being.

Flu- see Influenza

Fluke- a parasitic flatworm that can infest humans

Fluoride- a mineral that helps protect teeth against decay

Fluoroscopy- a method used to view organ structure and function by passing X-rays through the body and monitoring the resulting image on a fluorescent screen

Folic acid- a vitamin essential to the production of red blood cells; plays an important role in the growth a developing fetus

Follicle- a tiny pouchlike cavity in a structure of the body, such as a hair follicle

Follicle stimulating hormone- a hormone produced by the pituitary gland in the brain that stimulates the testicles to produce sperm in males and causes eggs to mature in females

Folliculitis- the inflammation of hair follicles due to a bacterial infection, causing boils or tiny blisters containing pus

Fontanelles- the two soft spots on a baby's scalp that are the result of gaps in the skull where bones have not yet fused

Food poisoning- stomach pain, diarrhea, and/or vomiting caused by eating contaminated food

Food poisoning- intoxicación alimentaria

Foot- pie

Forceps- instruments resembling tweezers that are used to handle objects or tissue during surgery

Forceps delivery- the use of an instrument that cups the baby's head (called an obstetric forceps), to help deliver a baby

Forearm- antebrazo

Foreign body- an object in an organ or body cavity that is not normally present

Foreskin- the loose skin that covers the head of the penis

Fracture- a bone break

Fracture- fractura

Fraternal twins- twins that develop from two different eggs fertilized by two different sperm; are not identical

Free radical- see Oxygen free radical

Frostbite- damage to body tissue as a result of freezing

FSH- see Follicle stimulating hormone

Fulminant- describes a disorder that begins suddenly and worsens quickly

Fungus- an organism that is dependent on another organism for nourishment

G

Galactocele- a milk-filled tumor in a blocked breast milk duct

Galactorrhea- breast milk production by a woman who is not pregnant and has not just given birth

Galactogogue- Stimulates the production or flow of breast milk in lactating women. They may act hormonally, or may include herbs that are nutritive, to improve milk quality and quantity

Galactose- a sugar that is formed from the breakdown of lactose

Galactosemia- a genetic disorder in which galactose cannot be converted into glucose

Gallbladder- a small, pear-shaped sac positioned under the liver, which concentrates and stores bile

Gallbladder- vesícula biliar

Gallstone- a round, hard mass of cholesterol, bile, or calcium salts that is found in the gallbladder or a bile duct

Gallstone ileus- an abnormal condition in which a gallstone passes from the gallbladder into the intestines through an abnormal passage and blocks the intestine

Gamete intrafallopian transfer- a method of treating infertility in which eggs are taken from a woman's ovaries and fertilized with sperm and then the fertilized egg is injected into one of her fallopian tubes

Gamma globulin- a substance prepared from blood that carries antibodies to most common infections; also used in immunizations

Ganglion- a fluid-filled cyst attached to a tendon sheath or joint

Gangrene- death of a tissue because of a lack of blood supply

Gastrectomy- surgical removal of all or part of the stomach

Gastric acid- the digestive acid in the stomach

Gastric juice- digestive fluids produced by the lining of the stomach that break down proteins and destroy harmful organisms

Gastric lavage- washing out of the stomach with water, often to treat poisoning; commonly called "stomach pumping"

Gastric ulcer- a peptic ulcer

Gastrin- a hormone that stimulates the release of gastric acid in the stomach

Gastrinoma- a tumor that produces gastrin, making the stomach and duodenum more acidic

Gastritis- inflammation of the mucous membrane lining of the stomach; can have a number of causes, including viruses, bacteria, and use of alcohol and other drugs

Gastroenteritis- inflammation of the stomach and intestines

Gastrointestinal series- a set of X-rays, taken at different intervals after a barium sulfate solution is swallowed, to examine the gastrointestinal tract

Gastrointestinal tract- the part of the digestive system that includes the mouth, esophagus, stomach, and intestines

Gastroscopy- examination of the esophagus, stomach, and the first part of the small intestine (duodenum) using an endoscope inserted through the mouth

Gastrostomy- the surgical creation of an opening in the abdominal wall into the stomach for drainage or a feeding tube

Gaucher's disease- a genetic disorder in which lipids cannot be properly broken down and build up in certain cells; causes enlargement of the spleen and liver, bone damage, and anemia

Gavage- an artificial feeding technique in which liquids are passed into the stomach by way of a tube inserted through the nose

Gene- the basic unit of DNA, which is responsible for passing genetic information; each gene contains the instructions for the production of a certain protein

General anesthesia- a method of preventing pain in which the patient is induced to lose consciousness

Generic drug- a drug marketed under its chemical name, instead of a brand name

Gene therapy- an experimental procedure in which disease-causing genes are replaced by normal, healthy genes

Genetic analysis- examination of DNA in a laboratory to diagnose genetic disorders

Genetic counseling- information and advice given to persons considering pregnancy about the risk that a child will have an inheritable birth defect or genetic disorder

Genetic disorder- a disorder caused partly or completely by a defect in genes, which carry hereditary information

Genetic engineering- the alteration of genetic information to change an organism; mainly used to produce vaccines and drugs such as insulin

Genital herpes- an infection caused by the herpes simplex virus, which causes a painful rash of fluid-filled blisters on the genitals; transmitted through sexual contact

Genital tract- the organs that make up the reproductive system

Genital wart- a growth on the skin in or around the vagina, penis, or anus, transmitted by sexual contact; can cause cancer of the cervix

Genome- the complete set of an organism's genes

Geographic tongue- a condition in which the tongue is patchy where surface cells break down

German measles- the common name for Rubella

Germ cell- a sperm or egg cell, or the immature form of either

Gestation- the period of time between fertilization of an egg by a sperm and birth of a baby

Gestational diabetes- is diabetes diagnosed for the first time during pregnancy.

Gestational hypertension- high blood pressure (over 140/90) that develops during pregnancy, but without evidence of kidney or liver damage.

to get hurt- lastimarse

Giardiasis- infection with a single-celled parasite, causing abdominal cramps, diarrhea, and nausea

GIFT- see Gamete intrafallopian transfer

Gingivectomy- surgical removal of a diseased part of the gums

Gingivitis- inflammation of the gums, typically caused by a buildup of plaque due to poor hygiene

GI series- see Gastrointestinal series

Gland- a group of cells or an organ that produces substances (such as hormones and

enzyme) that are used by the body

Glaucoma- a disease in which eye damage is caused by an increase in the pressure of the fluid within the eye

Glioblastoma multiforme- a fast-growing, cancerous brain tumor

Glioma- a brain tumor arising from cells that support nerve cells

Glomerulonephritis- inflammation of the filtering structures in the kidneys, hindering removal of waste products from the blood

Glomerulosclerosis- scarring of the filtering structures in the kidneys due to damage

Glossectomy- surgical removal of all or part of the tongue

Glucagon- a hormone produced by the pancreas that converts stored carbohydrates (glycogen) into glucose, the body's energy source

Glucose- a sugar that is the main source of energy for the body

Glucose tolerance test- a test that evaluates the body's response to glucose after a period of fasting; used to check for diabetes mellitus

Gluteus- gluteo

Glycogen- the main form that glucose, the body's energy source, takes when it is stored

Glycosuria- glucose in the urine

Goiter- enlargement of the thyroid gland, which produces a swelling on the neck

Gonadotropic hormones- hormones that stimulate activity in the ovaries and testicles

Gonorrhea- a common sexually transmitted disease, characterized by painful urination or a discharge from the penis or vagina

Gout- a disorder marked by high levels of uric acid in the blood; usually experienced as arthritis in one joint

Graft- healthy tissue that is used to replace diseased or defective tissue

Grand mal- a type of seizure occurring with epilepsy, producing loss of consciousness and involuntary jerking movements

Granuloma- a mass of tissue that forms at a site of inflammation, injury, or infection as a part of the healing process

Graves' disease- an autoimmune disease that causes goiter, overproduction of thyroid hormones, and sometimes bulging eyeballs

Guillain-Barré syndrome- a peripheral nervous system disease in which nerve inflammation causes weakness, loss of movement, and loss of sensation in the arms and legs

Guthrie test- a blood test performed on babies to test for phenylketonuria

Gynecologic examination- traditionally includes an examination of the external and internal genitalia (female). Under some conditions, it may be necessary to perform a rectal examination as well

H

Hair follicle- a tiny opening in the skin from which a hair grows

Halitosis- the clinical term for bad breath; commonly caused by poor oral hygiene or eating certain foods; if persistent it can be a sign of illness

Hallucination- a perception that occurs when there is actually nothing there to cause it (such as hearing voices when there are none)

Hammer toe- an abnormality in the tendons of the toe that causes the toe to be flexed at all times

Hamstring muscle- a muscle located at the back of the thigh that bends the leg at the knee and moves the leg backward

Hand- mano

Hardening of the arteries- the common name for arteriosclerosis

Hashimoto's disease- a disease in which the body's immune system attacks cells of the thyroid gland, resulting in a decrease in thyroid hormones

Hay fever- the common name for allergic rhinitis

HDL- see High-density lipoprotein

Head- cabeza

Headache- dolor de cabeza (pain in the head)

Heart- corazón

Heart attack- see Myocardial infarction

Heart attack- ataque al corazón /infarto de miocardio

Heart block- a disorder of the heart caused by a blockage of the nerve impulses to the heart that regulate heartbeat; may lead to dizziness, fainting, or stroke

Heartburn- a burning sensation experienced in the center of the chest up to the throat; may be caused by overeating, eating spicy food, or drinking alcohol; recurrent heartburn may be caused by acid reflux

Heart disease- see Coronary heart disease

Heart failure- the inability of the heart to pump blood effectively

Heart-lung machine- a machine that takes over the functions of the heart and lungs during certain types of surgery

Heart rate- the rate at which the heart pumps blood, measured in the number of heartbeats per minute

Heart valve- the structure at each exit of the four chambers of the heart that allows blood to exit but not to flow back in

Heat exhaustion- fatigue, dizziness, and nausea experienced because of overexposure to heat; if not treated it can result in heat stroke

Heat stroke- a life-threatening condition resulting from extreme overexposure to heat, which disrupts the body's system of regulating temperature

Heel spur- an abnormal, often painful outgrowth of bone on the back of the heel

Heimlich maneuver- a first-aid technique for choking; dislodges an object that is blocking a person's airway

Helper T cells- white blood cells, responsible for regulating other cells in the body's immune system, that are the main targets of the AIDS virus; also called CD4 cells

Hemangioma- a purple-red mark on the skin, caused by an excess of blood vessels

Hemarthrosis- bleeding into and swelling of a joint

Hematemesis- vomiting of blood

Hematocrit- the percentage of total blood volume that consists of red blood cells, which is determined by laboratory testing; can be an indicator of disease or injury

Hematoma- an accumulation of blood from a broken blood vessel

Hematuria- blood in the urine, which can be caused by urinary tract disorders (such as cysts, tumor, or stones) or by an infection

Hemochromatosis- a genetic disorder in which too much iron is absorbed from food

Hemodialysis- a method used to treat kidney failure, in which blood is passed through a machine that purifies it and returns it to the body

Hemoglobin- the pigment in red blood cells that is responsible for carrying oxygen; hemoglobin bound to oxygen gives blood its red color

Hemoglobinuria- hemoglobin in the urine

Hemolysis- the breakdown of red blood cells in the spleen, which is normal but can cause jaundice and anemia when the red blood cells are broken down too quickly

Hemophilia- an inherited disorder in which a person's blood lacks a certain protein important in forming blood clots, leading to excessive bleeding

Hemorrhage- the medical term for bleeding

Hemorrhage- hemorragia

Hemorrhoid- a bulging vein either at the opening of the anus or just inside the anus, often caused by childbirth or straining during bowel movements

Hemospermia- blood in the semen

Hemostasis- the stopping of bleeding by the body's mechanisms

Hemothorax- an accumulation of blood between the chest wall and the lungs

Hepatectomy- surgical removal of all or part of the liver

Hepatic- a term used to describe something that is related to the liver

Hepatitis- inflammation of the liver, which may be caused by a viral infection, poisons, or the use of alcohol or other drugs

Hepatitis A- a form of hepatitis caused by the hepatitis A virus, usually transmitted by contact with contaminated food or water

Hepatitis B- a form of hepatitis (generally more serious than hepatitis A) caused by the hepatitis B virus, which is transmitted through sexual contact or contact with infected blood or body fluids

Hepatitis C- a form of hepatitis caused by the hepatitis C virus, which is transmitted through sexual contact or contact with infected blood or body fluids

Hepatitis D- a form of hepatitis that only causes symptoms when the individual is already infected with hepatitis B

Hepatoma- a cancerous tumor of the liver

Hepatomegaly- enlargement of the liver

Herbalism- The art and science of using plants to nourish the body, mind, and spirit to support healing and promotion of well-being. Also encompasses ritualistic, folkloric, and cultural symbolism. Can include the use of whole plants or plant extracts in the form of foods, teas, powdered herbs, liquid extracts, incense, smudges, and skin preparations.

Hereditary- describes a genetic trait that is passed from parents to children

Hereditary spherocytosis- a genetic disorder in which red blood cells are smaller, rounder, and more fragile than normal, causing hemolytic anemia

Hermaphroditism- a rare condition in which an individual is born with both male and female reproductive organs

Hernia- the bulging of an organ or tissue through a weakened area in the muscle wall

Herniated disk- see Disk prolapse

Herpes encephalitis- brain inflammation caused by a herpes simplex virus that has spread from another part of the body

Herpes simplex- infection by the herpes simplex virus, which causes blisterlike sores on the face, lips, mouth, or genitals; in rare cases, can also affect the eyes, fingers, or brain

Herpes zoster- see Shingles

Heterosexuality- being sexually attracted to members of the opposite sex

Hiatal hernia- a type of hernia in which the stomach bulges up into the chest cavity through an opening in the diaphragm

Hiccup- involuntary sudden contraction of the diaphragm along with the closing of the vocal cords, producing a "hiccup" sound

High-density lipoprotein- a type of protein found in the blood that removes cholesterol from tissues, protecting against heart disease

High pressure- hipertensión arterial

High-tension- tensión alta

Hip- cadera

Hirschsprung's disease- a condition that is present at birth in which nerve cells do not develop in parts of the intestine, causing the intestine to narrow and block the passage of feces

Hirsutism- excessive hair or hair growth in unusual places, especially in women

Histamine- a chemical in some cells of the body that is released during allergic reactions, causing inflammation; also causes production of acid in the stomach and narrowing of the airways

H1 (histamine) blocker- a drug that blocks the action of histamine; used to treat inflammation

H2 (histamine) blocker- a drug used in the treatment of peptic ulcers that blocks histamine from causing acid production in the stomach

Histoplasmosis- a respiratory disease acquired by inhaling the spores of a fungus found in soil, especially where there are bird or bat droppings

HIV- see Human immunodeficiency virus

Hives- the common term for urticaria, an itchy, inflamed rash that results from an allergic

reaction

Hodgkin's disease- a cancer of lymphoid tissue (found in lymph nodes and the spleen) that causes the lymph nodes to enlarge and function improperly; may cause illness, fever, loss of appetite, and weight loss

Homeopathy- Based on the theory "like cures like," homeopathic preparations made of diluted plant, mineral, or animal substances are "matched to specific symptom pattern profiles of illness to stimulate the body's natural healing process" (American Botanical Council, 2016).

Homeostasis- the body's coordinated maintenance of the stable, internal environment by regulating blood pressure, blood sugar, body temperature, etc

Homocystinuria- a genetic disorder in which an enzyme deficiency causes a substance called homocystine to build up in the blood, leading to mental handicap and skeletal abnormalities

Homosexuality- being sexually attracted to members of the same sex

Hookworm- infestation by a small, round, blood-sucking parasite; commonly causes a rash on the foot, but can also cause cough, pneumonia, and anemia

Hormonal implant- surgical insertion of a small object just under the skin that slowly releases a synthetic hormone for purposes such as birth control

Hormone- a chemical produced by a gland or tissue that is released into the bloodstream; controls body functions such as growth and sexual development

Hormone replacement therapy- the use of natural or artificial hormones to treat hormone deficiencies

Hospice- a hospital or an area of a hospital dedicated to treating people who are dying, often of a specific cause

Hot flash- a sudden, temporary feeling of heat and sometimes sweating; usually occurs as a result of low estrogen levels in women because of menopause or after a hysterectomy

HTLV- see Human T-cell lymphotrophic virus

Human immunodeficiency virus- a retrovirus that attacks helper T cells of the immune system and causes acquired immunodeficiency syndrome (AIDS); transmitted through sexual intercourse or contact with infected blood

Human T-cell lymphotrophic virus- a virus similar to HIV that affects the same helper T cells, but usually accompanies adult T-cell leukemia or T-cell lymphomas

Hydramnios- an excess of amniotic fluid in the uterus during pregnancy

Hydrocele- a painless swelling of the scrotum, caused by a collection of fluid around the testicle; commonly occurs in middle aged men

Hydrocephalus- excess cerebrospinal fluid within the brain; commonly referred to as "water on the brain"

Hydrocortisone- a corticosteroid drug that is used to treat inflammation and allergies

Hygiene- the practice, maintenance, and study of health; commonly refers to cleanliness

Hymen- a thin fold of membrane partly closing the opening of the vagina; usually torn during first sexual intercourse or insertion of a tampon

Hyperactivity- a type of behavior characterized by excessive physical activity, sometimes associated with neurological or psychological causes

Hyperalimentation- a method of providing nutrients by the use of a tube or intravenously to a person who cannot eat food or needs nutrients because of an illness

Hyperbilirubinemia- a condition in which there is too much bilirubin, a substance produced when red blood cells are broken down; can lead to jaundice

Hypercalcemia- a condition marked by abnormally high levels of calcium in the blood; can lead to disturbance of cell function in the nerves and muscles and, if not treated, can be fatal

Hypercholesterolemia- an abnormally high level of cholesterol in the blood, which can be the result of an inherited disorder or a diet that is high in fat

Hyperglycemia- a condition characterized by abnormally high levels of glucose in the blood, usually as a result of untreated or improperly controlled diabetes mellitus

Hyperglycemia- hiperglucemia

Hyperlipidemia- a general term for a group of disorders in which lipid levels in the blood are abnormally high, including hypercholesterolemia

Hyperparathyroidism- overactivity of the parathyroid glands, which increases calcium levels in the blood (called hypercalcemia) and decreases calcium in bones (causing osteoporosis)

Hyperplasia- the enlargement of an organ or tissue

Hypersensitivity- an excessive response of the body's immune system to a foreign protein

Hypertension- abnormally high blood pressure, even when at rest

Hyperthermia- an abnormally high body temperature

Hyperthyroidism- overactivity of the thyroid gland, causing nervousness, weight loss, fatigue, and diarrhea

Hypertrophy- increase in the size of an organ due to an increase in the size of its cells Hyperventilation- abnormally rapid breathing

Hypochondriasis- an abnormal condition in which a person is overly concerned with health and believes that he or she is suffering from a major illness despite medical opinion to the contrary

Hypodermic needle- a thin, hollow needle attached to a syringe; used to inject a medication under the skin, into a vein, or into a muscle

Hypoglycemia- abnormally low levels of glucose in the blood
Hypoplasia- failure of a tissue or organ to develop normally

Hypoglycemia- hipoglucemia

Hypotension- the medical term for abnormally low blood pressure, which results in reduced blood flow to the brain, causing dizziness and fainting

Hypothermia- an abnormally low body temperature

Hypothyroidism- underactivity of the thyroid gland, causing tiredness, cramps, a slowed heart rate, and possibly weight gain

Hypoventilation- a slower-than-normal breathing rate

Hypoxemia- a reduced level of oxygen in the blood

Hypoxia- a reduced level of oxygen in tissues

Hysterectomy- surgical removal of the uterus

Hysteria- a term used to describe symptoms that are caused by mental stress and occur in someone who does not have a mental disorder

Hysterosalpingography- an X-ray examination performed to examine the inside of the uterus and fallopian tubes, in order to investigate and possibly treat infertility

Hysteroscopy- a method used to examine the inside of the uterus and the cervix using a viewing instrument

I

Iatrogenic- a term used to describe a disease, disorder, or medical condition that is a direct result of medical treatment

Itching- picazón

Ichthyosis- a variety of diseases in which the skin is dry and scaly

Idiopathic- a term used to describe something that occurs of an unknown cause

Ileostomy- a surgical procedure in which the lower part of the small intestine (the ileum) is cut and brought to an opening in the abdominal wall, where feces can be passed out of the body

Ileum- the lowest section of the small intestine, which attaches to the large intestine Ilium- one of the two bones that form the hip on either side of the body

Imaging- the technique of creating pictures of structures inside of the body using X-rays, ultrasound waves, or magnetic fields

Immune deficiency- impairment of the immune system, which reduces protection against infection and illness

Immune system- the cells, substances, and structures in the body that protect against infection and illness

Immunity- resistance to a specific disease because of the responses of the immune system

Immunization- the process of causing immunity by injecting antibodies or provoking the body to make its own antibodies against a certain microorganism

Immunocompromised- weakening of the body's immune system

Immunodeficiency- failure of the body's immune system to fight disease

Immunoglobin- proteins in blood and tissue fluids that help destroy microorganisms such as bacteria and viruses

Immunology- the study of the immune system, including how it functions and disorders that affect it

Immunomodulant- Tonifies and strengthens the immune system.

Immunostimulant- a drug that increases the ability of the body's immune system to fight disease

Immunosuppressant- a drug that inhibits the activity of the immune system; used to prevent rejection of a transplant organ and in disorders where the body's immune system attacks its own tissues

Impacted fracture- a bone break in which the two broken ends have been forced into each other

Imperforate anus- a birth defect in which the opening of the anus is not formed normally

Impetigo- a highly contagious skin infection caused by bacteria, usually occurring around the nose and mouth; commonly occurring in children

Implant- an organ, tissue, or device surgically inserted and left in the body

Impotence- the inability to acquire or maintain an erection of the penis

Incompetent cervix- an abnormally weak cervix, which widens prematurely during pregnancy as a result of the weight of a developing fetus; may result in a miscarriage

Incontinence- inability to hold urine or feces inside of the body

Incubation period- the time period between when an infectious organism enters the body and when symptoms occur

Indigenous or Tribal Medicine- Refers to beliefs and practices related to care of the physical and spiritual being that have been passed generationally through oral tradition, ceremonies and rituals (American Botanical Council, 2016). Techniques may include use of botanical or animal medicine, prayer, ceremony, and ritual and are unique to each group, region, or tribe.

Indigestion- uncomfortable symptoms brought on by overeating or eating spicy, rich, or fatty foods; characterized by heartburn, pain in the abdomen, nausea, and gas, and can be more serious if recurrent

Induction of labor- the use of artificial means to start the process of childbirth Infarction- tissue death due to lack of blood supply

Infection- disease-causing microorganisms that enter the body, multiply, and damage cells or release toxins

Infection- infección

Infective arthritis- arthritis caused by bacteria from a wound or the bloodstream entering a joint

Infertility- the inability to have children as a result of sexual intercourse

Inflammation- redness, pain, and swelling in an injured or infected tissue produced as a result of the body's healing response

Inflammation / swelling- inflamación

Inflammatory bowel disease- the general term for two inflammatory disorders affecting the intestines; also known as Crohn's disease and ulcerative colitis

Inflammatory joint disease- any type of arthritis that causes a joint to become inflamed

Influenza- a viral infection characterized by headaches, muscle aches, fever, weakness, and cough; commonly called the "flu"

Informed consent- agreement to undergo a medical procedure after the technique, its risks, and its possible complications have been explained

Infusion- the introduction of a substance, such as a drug or nutrient, into the bloodstream or a body cavity

Infusion- A shorter (1-10 minute) water extraction of an herb typically used for softer plant parts such as leaves and flowers. May also be referred to as a tisane or tea

Infused Oil- An oil into which constituents or qualities of an herb have been imparted by infusion over a length of time from hours to several weeks, sometimes by applying heat.

Ingestion- taking something into the body through the mouth

Ingrown toenail- a painful condition of the big toe in which the nail grows into the skin on either side, causing inflammation and/or infection

Inguinal hernia- the bulging of a portion of the intestines or abdominal tissue into the muscles of the groin (the area just below the abdomen)

Inhaler- a device used to introduce a powdered or misted drug into the lungs through the mouth, usually to treat respiratory disorders such as asthma

Inheritance- the passing of traits from parent to child through genes

Injection- the use of a syringe and needle to insert a drug into a vein, muscle, or joint or under the skin

Injury/wound- lesión

Insemination- the placement of semen into a woman's uterus, cervix, or vagina

In situ- "in place"; often describes a cancer that has not spread

Insomnia- difficulty falling or remaining asleep

Insulin- a hormone made in the pancreas that plays an important role in the absorption of glucose (the body's main source of energy) into muscle cells

Insulin- insulina

Insulinoma- a noncancerous tumor of the insulin-producing cells of the pancreas; the tumor releases excess insulin into the blood, causing glucose levels to drop dangerously low

Intensive care- close monitoring of a patient who is seriously ill

Interferon- a protein produced by body cells that fights viral infections and certain cancers

Internal bleeding- bleeding inside the body, particularly in the chest cavity, belly cavity, or muscles, that may be caused by major trauma

Internal bleeding- hemorragia interna

Internal fixation- a method of holding a broken bone in place using surgically inserted screws, rods, or plates

Interstitial- lying between body structures or in the interspaces of tissues Interstitial cystitis- persistent inflammation of the lining and muscle of the bladder

Interstitial lung disease- a disease of the connective tissue surrounding the air sacs of the lungs that causes a dry cough, scarring of lung tissue, and shortness of breath

Interstitial pulmonary fibrosis- scarring of connective tissue in the lungs that leads to shortness of breath

Interstitial radiation therapy- a treatment for cancer in which a radioactive material is inserted into or near a tumor to provide direct radiation

Intervertebral disks- broad, flat cartilage structures containing a gel-like fluid that cushion and separate vertebrae

Intestinal bypass- a surgical procedure in which the beginning of the large intestine is joined to its end so that less food is absorbed; because of serious side effects, usually performed only on seriously obese people

Intestine- a long, tube-shaped organ that extends from the stomach to the anus; absorbs food and water and passes the waste products of digestion as feces

Intra-aortic balloon pump- a small balloon inserted into the aorta that helps to circulate blood by inflating between heartbeats

Intractable- describes a condition that does not respond to treatment

Intramedullary rod- a strong metal rod that is placed inside of a broken bone to help it heal correctly

Intraocular pressure- the pressure of the fluids within the eye

Intrauterine device- a device inserted into the uterus that helps to prevent pregnancy

Intravenous- inside of or into a vein

Intrinsic- a term used to describe something originating from or located in a tissue or organ

Intubation- the passage of a tube into an organ or body structure; commonly used to refer to the passage of a tube down the windpipe for artificial respiration

Invasive- describes something that spreads throughout body tissues, such as a tumor or microorganism; also describes a medical procedure in which body tissues are penetrated

In vitro- "in glass"; a biological test or process that is carried out in a laboratory

In vitro fertilization- a treatment for infertility in which an egg and a sperm are joined outside the woman's body, and the fertilized egg is then inserted into the uterus or fallopian tube

In vivo- "in the living body"; a biological process that occurs inside of the body

Involuntary- occurring without a person's control or participation

Iodine- an element for the formation of thyroid hormones

Ionizing radiation- radiation that damages cells or genes; can be used to treat cancer

IQ- intelligence quotient; a measure of a person's intelligence as determined by specific tests

Iris- the colored part of the eye

Iron- a mineral necessary for the formation of important biological substances such as hemoglobin, myoglobin, and certain enzymes

Iron-deficiency anemia- a type of anemia caused by a greater-than-normal loss of iron due to bleeding, problems absorbing iron, or a lack of iron in the diet

Irrigation- the cleansing of a wound by flushing it with water, a medicated solution, or some other fluid

Irritable bladder- involuntary contractions of muscles in the bladder, which can cause lack of control of urination

Irritable bowel syndrome- abnormal muscle movement in the intestines, which causes abdominal pain and irregular bowel movements (diarrhea, constipation, or both)

Irritation- irritación

Ischemia- a condition in which a tissue or organ does not receive a sufficient supply of blood

IUD- see Intrauterine device IVF- see In vitro fertilization

J

Jaundice- yellowing of the skin and whites of the eyes because of the presence of excess bilirubin in the blood; usually a sign of a disorder of the liver

Jock itch- an infection in the groin area caused by a fungus

Juvenile rheumatoid arthritis- a rare form of persistent joint inflammation that affects children

K

Kaposi's sarcoma- a skin cancer that is characterized by purple-red tumors that start at the feet and spread upward on the body; commonly occurs in people who have AIDS

Kawasaki disease- a childhood disease causing fever, rash, skin peeling, swollen lymph nodes, and possibly complications of the heart and brain

Keloid- a raised, firm, thick scar that forms as a result of a defect in the natural healing process

Keratin- a tough protein found in skin, nails, and hair Keratitis- inflammation of the cornea

Keratolytic- drugs that remove the keratin-containing outer layer of skin; used to treat skin disorders such as warts and dandruff

Keratoplasty- surgical replacement or reshaping of the cornea
Keratosis- a growth on the skin that is the result of overproduction of the protein keratin

Ketoacidosis- the dangerous accumulation of chemicals called ketones in the blood, sometimes occurring as a complication of diabetes mellitus; also called ketosis

Kidney- one of two organs that are part of the urinary tract; responsible for filtering the blood and removing waste products and excess water as urine

Kidney- riñón

Kidney stone- a hard mass composed of substances from the urine that form in the kidneys

Killer T cells- white blood cells that are part of the immune system and destroy microorganisms and cancer cells

Kilocalorie- a unit of energy; equal to a nutritional calorie

Kimmelstiel-Wilson syndrome- a kidney disorder that can occur as a complication of diabetes mellitus; can cause swelling, high blood pressure, and kidney failure

Klinefelter's syndrome- a genetic disorder in which a man has at least 1 extra X chromosome in his cells, causing infertility and female characteristics

Knee-jerk reflex- a test for a reflexive extension of the leg to check the functioning of the nervous system; tapping the knee just below the kneecap should cause the lower part of the leg to jerk upward

Kyphosis- excessive curvature of the spine, which usually affects the top part of the spine and causes a hump

L

Labia- the two pairs of skinfolds that protect the opening of the vagina

Labor- the interval from onset of contractions to birth of a baby

Labyrinthitis- inflammation of the fluid-containing chamber of the inner ear (called the labyrinth) that maintains balance; can cause a feeling that one's surroundings are spinning around (known as vertigo)

Laceration- a torn or ragged wound

Lactase deficiency- an inherited disorder in which a person does not have the enzyme lactase, which breaks down lactose (the sugar found in dairy products); lactase deficiency leads to lactose intolerance, which means the inability to digest lactose

Lactation- the production of breast milk after giving birth

Lactation suppression- a decrease in milk production during pregnancy as a result of high levels of estrogen in the blood

Lactic acid- an acid produced by glucose-burning cells when these cells have an insufficient supply of oxygen

Lactose- the sugar found in dairy products

Lactose intolerance- inability to break down and absorb the sugar lactose

Lamaze method- a method of preparing for childbirth that stresses physical conditioning, relaxation, and breathing exercises

Laminectomy- a surgical procedure that removes part of a vertebra to relieve pressure on the spinal cord or a nerve branching from the spinal cord

Laparoscope- a viewing instrument used to examine and treat disorders in the abdominal cavity; consists of a long tube with an eyepiece, a lens, and often a camera, which allows the image to be viewed on a monitor

Laparoscopic cholecystectomy- surgical removal of the gallbladder using a laparoscope

Laparoscopy- a procedure done to examine the abdominal cavity using a laparoscope,

usually to investigate pelvic pain or gynecologic conditions such as infertility

Large-cell carcinoma- one of the 4 major types of lung cancer

Large intestine- the part of the digestive tract that is located between the small intestine and the anus

Large intestine- intestino grueso

Laryngectomy- surgical removal of all or part of the voice box (larynx) as a treatment for cancer

Laryngitis- inflammation of the voice box, usually caused by a viral infection; characterized by a hoarse voice

Larynx- the medical term for the voice box, the organ in the throat that produces voice and also prevents food from entering the airway

Laser treatment- the use of a laser (a concentrated beam of light) to perform medical procedures, such as the destruction of tumors

Latent infection- an infection that lies dormant in the body for months or years but can reappear

Lateral- on one side

Laxatives- drugs used to clear feces from the intestines; commonly used to treat constipation

Lazy eye- the common name for the visual defect resulting from untreated strabismus, in which the eyes are not correctly aligned

LDL- see Low-density lipoprotein

Lead poisoning- damage to the brain, nerves, red blood cells, or digestive system because of ingestion of lead

Learning disability- any of a variety of disorders, including hyperactivity, dyslexia, and hearing problems, that can interfere with a person's ability to learn

Leg- pierna

Legionnaires 'disease- a form of pneumonia that is mainly spread through air- conditioning systems and water

Leiomyoma- a noncancerous tumor of smooth muscle

Leishmaniasis- a group of parasitic diseases affecting the skin, mucous membranes, and internal organs; transmitted by the bite of a sandfly

Leptospirosis- infection by a spiral-shaped bacterium that affects the skin, eyes, muscles, kidneys, and liver; leptospirosis is carried by rodents

Lesch-Nyhan syndrome- a genetic disorder affecting only men that causes mental handicap, self-mutilation, and aggressive behavior

Lesion- an abnormality of structure or function in the body

Leukemia- a group of bone marrow cancers in which white blood cells divide uncontrollably, affecting the production of normal white blood cells, red blood cells, and platelets

Leukocyte- another name for a white blood cells

Leukocyte count- the number of white blood cells in the blood, which is used as a measure of health and possible infection

Leukodystrophy- a group of childhood genetic disorders in which the protective coverings of the nerves are destroyed

Leukoplakia- white patches that can develop in the mouth or on the penis or the opening of the vagina and are potentially cancerous

LH- see Luteinizing hormone

Lichen planus- a common skin disease in which itchy, small, pink or purple spots appear on the arms or legs

Ligament- a tough, elastic band of tissue that connects bones and suupports organs Ligation- the process of closing a blood vessel or duct by tying it off

Liniment- A topical preparation typically prepared by infusing plants into alcohol.

Lipid-lowering drugs- drugs taken to lower the levels of specific fats called lipids in the blood in order to reduce the risk of narrowing of the arteries

Lipidosis- any disorder in which fats cannot be properly broken down by the digestive system

Lipids- a group of fats stored in the body and used for energy

Lipoma- a noncancerous tumor of fatty tissue

Lipoproteins- substances containing lipids and proteins, comprising most fats in the blood

Liposarcoma- a cancerous tumor of fatty tissue

Liposuction- a surgical procedure in which fat is removed from areas of the body using a suction pump

Listeriosis- a rare bacterial infection acquired by eating undercooked infected meat or from infected live animals; can be dangerous to newborns and the elderly

Lithotripsy- a procedure done to break up stones in the urinary tract using ultrasonic shock waves, so that the fragments can be easily passed from the body

Liver- the largest organ in the body, producing many essential chemicals and regulating the levels of most vital substances in the blood

Liver- hígado

Liver failure- the final stage of liver disease, in which liver function becomes so impaired that other areas of the body are affected, most commonly the brain

Lobe- a well-defined, separate part of an organ

Lobectomy- surgical removal of a lobe

Local anesthesia- a method of preventing pain by inducing the loss of sensation in a certain area of the body while the patient remains awake

Locked joint- a joint that cannot be moved because of a disease or a lodged piece of bone or cartilage

Lockjaw- a spasm of the jaw muscles that prevents the mouth from opening, such as that caused by tetanus

Locomotor system- the structures of the body that are responsible for its movement

Lordosis- the inward curvature of the spine at the lower back, which is normal to a certain degree; abnormal as a result of certain medical conditions, being overweight, or having muscle problems

Lou Gehrig's disease- see Amyotrophic lateral sclerosis

Low-density lipoprotein- a type of lipoprotein that is the major carrier of cholesterol in the blood, with high levels associated with narrowing of the arteries and heart disease

Lower back pain- dolor lumbar

Low pressure- hipotensión arterial

Lumbago- dull, aching pain in the lower back

Lumbar puncture- a procedure in which a needle is inserted into the lower region of the spinal canal to take out a sample of spinal fluid or to inject a drug

Lumbar spine- the lower part of the spine between the lowest pair of ribs and the pelvis; made up of five vertebrae

Lumpectomy- surgical removal of a section of breast containing cancer

Lung collapse- a condition in which all or part of a lung cannot expand and fill with air

Lungs- two organs in the chest that take in oxygen from the air and release carbon dioxide

Lungs- pulmones

Lupus erythematosus- a disorder of the immune system that causes inflammation of connective tissue

Luteinizing hormone- a hormone produced by the pituitary gland that causes the ovaries and testicles to release sex hormones and plays a role in the development of eggs and sperm

Lyme disease- a disease caused by bacteria transmitted through the bite of a tick; characterized by fever, rash, and inflammation of the heart and joints

Lymph- a milky fluid containing white blood cells, proteins, and fats; plays an important role in absorbing fats from the intestine and in the functioning of the immune system

Lymphadenopathy- swollen lymph nodes

Lymphangiography- an X-ray procedure that creates images of the lymphatic system Lymphatic system- a network of vessels that drain lymph back into the blood

Lymph node- a small gland that is part of the immune system; contains white blood cells and antibodies and helps fight against the spread of infection

a **Lymphatic**- Aids in movement of lymph through the lymphatic system.

Lymphocyte- a white blood cell that is an important part of the body's immune system, helping to destroy invading microorganisms

Lymphocytic leukemia- a disease in which white blood cells called lymphocytes divide uncontrollably

Lymphogranuloma venereum- a sexually transmitted chlamydial infection; common in countries with a tropical climate

Lymphomas- a group of cancer of the lymph nodes and spleen that can spread to other parts of the body

Lymphosarcoma- another name for a non-Hodgkin's sarcoma; a cancerous tumor in lymphoid tissue

M

Maceration- A liquid extract prepared by combining herbs with a solvent such as ethanol, vinegar, or vegetable glycerine.

Macula- the area of the retina that allows fine details to be observed at the center of vision; also refers to any small, flat spot on the skin

Macular degeneration- gradual loss of vision due to deterioration of nerve tissue in the retina

Magnesium- a mineral that is essential for many body functions, including nerve impulse transmission, formation of bones and teeth, and muscle contraction

Magnetic resonance imaging (MRI)- a technique that uses magnetic fields and radio waves to create high-quality cross-sectional images of the body without using radiation

Malabsorption- an impaired ability of the lining of the small intestine to absorb nutrients from food

Malaria- a parasitic disease spread by mosquitos that causes chills and fever; potentially fatal complications in the liver, kidneys, blood, and brain are possible

Malformation- abnormal development of an organ or tissue

Malignant- a word used to describe a condition that is characterized by uncontrolled growth and/or that can be fatal, such as a cancerous tumor

Malignant hyperthermia- a reaction to certain anesthesia gases involving intense muscle contractions and a high fever

Malignant melanoma- the most serious type of skin cancer, in which a mole changes shape, darkens, becomes painful, and/or bleeds easily

Mallory-Weiss syndrome- a condition associated with alcoholism in which the lower end of the esophagus tears, causing vomiting of blood

Mammography- an X-ray procedure done to detect breast cancer

Mammoplasty- a general term for a cosmetic operation on the breasts; includes breast reduction, enlargement, and reconstruction after a mastectomy

Mandible- another term for the lower jaw

Mania- a mental disorder characterized by extreme excitement, happiness, overactivity, and agitation; usually refers to the high of the highs and lows experienced in manic-depressive disorder

Manic-depressive disorder- a mental disorder characterized by extreme mood swings, including either mania, depression, or a continuing shift between the two extremes

MAO inhibitor- see Monoamine oxidase inhibitor antidepressant

Marc- The solid plant or mushroom component of the tincture or extract making process.

Marfan's syndrome- a rare genetic disorder that affects connective tissue, leading to abnormalities of joints, bones, tendons, ligaments, arteries, and/or the heart

Mast cell- a type of cell present in most body tissues that releases substances in response to an allergen, which causes symptoms such as inflammation

Mastectomy- a surgical procedure in which all or part of the breast is removed to prevent the spread of cancer

Mastitis- inflammation of the breast, which is usually caused by a bacterial infection

Maxilla- one of two bones that form the upper jaw, the roof of the mouth, and the center portion of the face

Measles- an illness caused by a viral infection, causing a characteristic rash and a fever; primarily affects children

Meconium- thick, sticky, greenish-brown stool passed by a postmature fetus, or one experiencing fetal distress, into the amniotic fluid, or by an infant during the first couple of days after birth

Medial- a term used to describe something situated on or near the midline of the body or a body structure

Median nerve- a nerve running down the arm to the hand; controls muscle movement in the forearm and hand and conveys sensation from part of the hand

Mediastinoscopy- investigation of the central chest compartment using an endoscope that is inserted through an incision in the neck

Medulla- the center part of an organ or body structure; sometimes used to refer to the lower part of the brain stem

Medulloblastoma- a type of cancerous tumor, occurring in the section of the brain that controls posture and balance; found mainly in children

Megacolon- a severely swollen large intestine, causing severe constipation and abdominal bloating; may be present at birth or develops later

Megaloblastic anemia- a type of anemia in which a lack of the vitamin B12 or folic acid interferes with red blood cells and causes them to be enlarged and deformed, resulting in tiredness and weight loss

Meiosis- the type of cell division that occurs only in the ovaries and testicles, producing cells with half the genes of the original cell; these cells then form eggs and sperm

Melanin- the pigment that gives skin, hair, and eyes their coloring

Melanocytes- cells that produce the pigment melanin

Melanocyte-stimulating hormone- a hormone that coordinates pigmentation of the skin, eyes, and hair

Melanoma- a skin tumor composed of cells called melanocytes

Memory loss- pérdida de memoria

Menarche- the beginning of menstruation

Meniere's disease- a disorder of the inner ear, causing hearing loss, ringing in the ear, and the sensation that one's surroundings are spinning

Meninges- the three membranes that surround and protect the spinal cord and brain

Meningioma- a rare noncancerous tumor developing in the protective membranes covering the brain called the meninges; can cause headaches and problems with vision and mental function

Meningitis- inflammation of the meninges; usually caused by infection by a microorganism (meningitis caused by bacteria is life-threatening; viral meningitis is milder)

Meningocele- a protrusion of the meninges through an opening in the skull or spinal cord due to a genetic defect

Meniscectomy- surgical removal of all or part of a cartilage disk from a joint Meniscus- a crescent-shaped pad of cartilage in joints that helps to reduce friction

Menopause- the period in a woman's life when menstruation stops, resulting in a reduced production of estrogen and cessation of egg production

Menorrhagia- excessive loss of blood during menstruation, which can be caused by disorders of the uterus

Menstrual cycle- the periodic discharge of blood and mucosal tissue from the uterus, occurring from puberty to menopause in a woman who is not pregnant

Menstruation- the shedding of the lining of the uterus during the menstrual cycle Mesenteric infarction- death of tissue in the intestine due to lack of blood supply to that tissue

Menstruum- The liquid component of a tincture making process, e.g., alcohol, vinegar, or glycerine.

Mesenteric lymphadenitis- inflammation of lymph nodes in an abdominal membrane

Mesothelioma- a cancerous tumor occurring in the lining of the lungs and chest cavity, often associated with exposure to asbestos dust

Mesothelium- a tissue layer that lines the heart, abdomen, chest cavity, and lungs

Messenger RNA- an RNA molecule that transports the information stored in DNA out of a cell's nucleus in order to make proteins

Metabolic rate- the speed at which the body uses energy

Metabolism- a general term for all of the chemical processes that occur in the body

Metabolite- any substance that takes part in a chemical reaction in the body

Metastasis- the spreading of a cancerous tumor to another part of the body through lymph, blood, or across a cavity; also sometimes refers to a tumor that has been produced in this way

Metered-dose inhaler- an inhaler that gives a specific amount of medication with each use

Metformin- metformina

Microbe- another term for a microorganism, especially one that causes disease

Microbe- microbio

Microbiology- the study of microorganisms

Microcephaly- an abnormally small head

Microdiskectomy- surgical removal of the protruding part of a prolapsed disk

Microorganism- any tiny, single-celled organism (such as a bacterium, virus, or fungus)

Microsurgery- a surgical technique that uses a special binocular microscope to operate on tiny, delicate, or hard-to-reach tissues

Micturition syncope- fainting or feeling weak while standing at the toilet; caused by an abnormal heartbeat or a drop in blood pressure

Middle ear- the small cavity between the eardrum and inner ear; contains three tiny, linked bones that transmit sound to the inner ear

Middle ear effusion- the buildup of fluid in the middle ear, which can affect hearing

Midwifery- a profession concerned with providing care to a mother and baby during pregnancy and childbirth

Migraine- a severe headache, usually accompanied by vision problems and/or nausea and vomiting, and that typically recurs

Mineral- a substance that is a necessary part of a healthy diet (such as potassium, calcium, sodium, phosphorus, and magnesium)

Minipill- an oral contraceptive containing only the synthetic hormone progesterone (birth control pills contain estrogen and progesterone)

Miotic- a drug that causes the pupil to constrict

Miscarriage- expulsion of a fetus before it has developed sufficiently to survive on its own

Mites- small eight-legged animals, many of which burrow and feed on blood

Mitosis- the process by which most cells divide in order to reproduce

Mitral insufficiency- a problem with the ability of the mitral valve in the heart to close, which causes the heart to pump harder and reduces its efficiency

Mitral stenosis- a condition in which the mitral valve in the heart becomes narrowed, making the heart work harder to pump blood; can lead to symptoms such as shortness of breath

Mitral valve- the valve in the heart that allows blood to flow from the left atrium to the left ventricle, but prevents blood from flowing back in

Mitral valve prolapse- a common condition in which the mitral valve in the heart is deformed, causing blood to leak back across the valve; characterized by a heart murmur and sometimes chest pain and disturbed heart rhythm

Modified radical mastectomy- a treatment for breast cancer in which the entire breast, a section of the chest muscle, and lymph nodes in the chest and underarm are removed

Molar tooth- large, strong teeth at the back of the jaw, primarily used to grind food

Mole- a brown to dark-brown spot on the skin that can be flat or raised

Molecule- the smallest unit of a substance that possesses its characteristics

Molluscum contagiosum- a viral infection that causes white bumps on the skin; usually clears up in a few months

Mongolian spot- a brown to blue-black spot on the lower back and buttocks at birth, caused by a concentration of pigment-producing cells; usually disappears by the age of 3 or 4 years

Monoamine oxidase inhibitor antidepressant- a substance that works by stopping an enzyme that breaks down stimulating chemicals in the brain; used to treat depression

Monoclonal antibodies- an antibody that is produced in the laboratory so that it will react with only one specific foreign protein; used to help diagnose certain kinds of cancer

Mononucleosis- an infection caused by a virus that invades a type of white blood cell called a monocyte, causing fever, sore throat, and swollen lymph nodes

Monounsaturated fat- a type of fat that is thought to be beneficial in the prevention of coronary heart disease; found in foods such as olive oil and peanut oil

Morbidity- the state of being ill or having a disease

Morning sickness- nausea and vomiting experienced early in a pregnancy, affecting about half of all pregnant women

Mortality- the death rate, measured as the number of deaths per a certain population; may describe the population as a whole, or a specific group within a population (such as infant mortality)

Motor nerve- a nerve that carries messages to a muscle that cause the muscle to contract

Motor neuron disease- degeneration of the nerves in the spinal cord and brain that are responsible for muscle movement, causing weakness and muscle deterioration

Mouth- boca

Mouth-to-mouth resuscitation- a method of artificial breathing in which someone rhythmically forces air into the lungs of a person who has stopped breathing

MRI- see Magnetic resonance imaging

MS- see Multiple sclerosis

Mucocele- a sac or body cavity that is swollen because of the production of mucus by the cells in its lining

Mucolytic- a drug that lessens the sticky quality of phlegm and makes it easier to cough up

Mucous membrane- the soft, pink layer of cells that produce mucus in order to keep body structures lubricated; found in structures such as the eyelids, respiratory tract, and urinary tract

Mucus- a slippery fluid produced by mucous membranes that lubricates and protects the internal surfaces of the body

Multi-infarct dementia- dementia caused by multiple strokes

Multiple-gated acquisition scan- a technique for evaluating heart efficiency by measuring blood flow into and out of the heart

Multiple myeloma- a cancer that causes uncontrolled production of white blood cells in the bone marrow

Multiple pregnancy- the presence of more than one fetus in the uterus, such as occurs with twins

Multiple sclerosis- a disease in which the protective coverings (myelin) of nerve fibers in the brain are gradually destroyed; symptoms vary from numbness to paralysis and loss of control of bodily function

Mumps- a viral infection that causes inflammation of salivary glands; primarily affects children

Murmur- a characteristic sound (heard through a stethoscope) of blood flowing irregularly through the heart; can be harmless or may be an indication of disease

Muscle- músculo

Muscle fibers- specialized, contracting cells that are bundled together to form muscles

Muscle relaxants- a group of drugs used to relieve muscle spasm and to treat conditions such as arthritis, back pain, and nervous system disorders such as stroke and cerebral palsy

Muscle tone- the natural tension in resting muscles

Muscle wasting- the degeneration of a muscle (loss of bulk), caused by disease or starvation

Muscular dystrophy- a rare genetic disorder in which muscles degenerate gradually and strength is lost

Mutagen- anything that can increase the rate of abnormal change in cells, which can lead to cancer

Mutation- a change in the genetic information within a cell

Myalgia- the medical term for muscle pain

Myasthenia gravis- a disease in which the muscles, mainly those in the face, eyes, throat, and limbs, become weak and tire quickly; caused by the body's immune system attacking the receptors in the muscles that pick up nerve impulses

Mycobacterium- a type of slow-growing bacterium; resistant to the body's defense mechanisms and are responsible for diseases such as tuberculosis and leprosy

Mycoplasma- the smallest free-living microorganisms

Mycosis- any disease caused by a fungus

Mydriatic- a drug that causes the pupil to dilate (widen)

Myelin sheath- the fat- and protein-containing material that surrounds and protects some nerves

Myelitis- inflammation of the spinal cord, which can cause headaches, fever, muscle stiffness, pain, weakness, and eventually paralysis

Myelocele- protrusion of the spinal cord and its coverings out from the spine; one of the more severe forms of spina bifida

Myeloma- a cancer affecting cells in the bone marrow; sometimes used as an abbreviation for multiple myeloma

Myelosclerosis- buildup of fibrous connective tissue in the bone marrow, affecting the production of blood components

Myocardial infarction- the death of an area of heart muscle as a result of being deprived of its blood supply; characterized by severe pain in the chest; commonly called a heart attack

Myocarditis- inflammation of the heart muscle, which can be caused by a virus, certain drugs, or radiation therapy

Myocarditis- miocarditis

Myocardium- the medical term for heart muscle

Myomectomy- the surgical removal of a noncancerous tumor from muscle

Myopathy- a muscle disease, usually one that results in the deterioration of muscle Myopia- the medical term for nearsightedness

Myositis- muscle inflammation, causing pain and weakness

Myringotomy- a surgical opening in the eardrum that allows for drainage

Myxoma- a noncancerous tumor made of mucous material and fibrous connective tissue

N

Narcolepsy- a disorder that causes excessive sleepiness during the day and frequent and uncontrollable episodes of falling asleep

Narcosis- a drug (or other chemical)-induced drowsiness or stupor

Narcotic- an addictive substance that blunts the senses; can cause confusion, stupor, coma, and death with increased dosages

Narcotic analgesics- a type of painkiller that blocks the transmission of pain signals in the brain; often cause tolerance (the need for higher amounts of the drug to produce the same effect) and drug dependence

Nasal septum- the section of the nose that divides the left and right nostrils; made of cartilage and bone and covered by a mucous membrane

Nasogastric tube- a thin, plastic tube that is inserted through the nose, down the esophagus, and into the stomach; used to drain, wash, or take samples from the stomach, or to feed very sick patients who cannot eat

Nasopharynx- the passageway connecting the back of the nose to the top of the throat

Natural childbirth- a technique of giving birth that stresses relaxation techniques so that the use of pain-relieving drugs can be minimized; also called prepared childbirth

Natural methods of family planning- methods of planning a family that focus on a woman's time of ovulation, either so that pregnancy can be avoided or conception is likely

Naturopathic Medicine-" Emphasizing prevention, treatment, and optimal health through the use of therapeutic methods and substances that encourage individuals 'inherent self-healing process" naturopathy "includes modern and traditional, scientific, and empirical methods" (American Association of Naturopathic Physicians, 2017). In the United States, twenty states license naturopathy. Currently, in the United States and Canada seven accredited naturopathic medical schools train Naturopathic Doctors who may apply for an ND license upon completion.

Nausea- feeling the need to vomit

Nebulizer- an instrument that provides a drug in its misted form through a face mask; used for severe asthma attacks and for children who have asthma but cannot use an inhaler

Neck- cuello

Necrosis- the medical term for the death of tissue cells

Needle aspiration- the use of a thin, hollow needle and syringe to remove body fluid for examination

Needle biopsy- the use of a hollow, wide-diameter needle to remove a sample of tissue for examination

Neonate- a term used to describe a newborn infant from birth to 1 month of age

Neoplasm- another term for a tumor

Nephrectomy- the surgical removal of one or both kidneys

Nephritis- inflammation of one or both kidneys because of an infection, an abnormal immune system response, or a disorder of metabolism

Nephroblastoma- a fast-growing cancer of the kidneys that occurs most commonly in children under 4 years of age

Nephrolithotomy- surgical removal of a kidney stone

Nephrons- the tiny filtering units of the kidney

Nephrosclerosis- the replacement of normal kidney structures with scar tissue

Nephrostomy- the surgical placement of a tube into the kidney to drain urine

Nephrotic syndrome- symptoms that result from damage to the filtering units of the kidney

Nerve- a bundle of fibers that transmit electrical messages between the brain and areas of the body; these messages convey sensory or motor function information

Nerve block- the dulling of sensation in an area of the body by injecting a painkiller into or around a nerve leading to that section of the body

Nerve cell- the basic unit of the nervous system; transmits chemical messages throughout the body

Nerve compression- pressure on a nerve, which can cause nerve damage and muscle weakness

Nervine- Herbs rich in volatile oils that have a beneficial effect on the nervous system, acting as a stimulant, sedative, or tonic.

Neuralgia- pain along the course of a nerve caused by irritation or damage to the nerve

Neural tube- the tube located along the back of an embryo that later develops into the spinal cord and brain

Neural tube defects- problems in the development of the spinal cord and brain in an embryo, such as the failure of the spine to enclose the spinal cord (spina bifida) and the failure of the brain to develop (anencephaly)

Neuritis- inflammation of a nerve, often characterized by pain, numbness, or tingling; also used to describe nerve damage and disease from causes other than inflammation

Neuroblastoma- a cancerous childhood tumor located in the adrenal glands or the sympathetic nervous system

Neurofibrillary tangles- abnormal spiral filaments on nerve cells in the brain; characteristic of Alzheimer disease

Neurofibromatosis- a condition in which connective tissue tumors occur on nerves in the skin

Neuroleptic- an antipsychotic drug

Neurological therapy- terapia neurológica

Neuroma- a noncancerous tumor occurring in nerve tissue

Neuron- another term for a nerve cell

Neuropathy- disease, inflammation, or damage to the nerves connecting the brain and spinal cord to the rest of the body

Neurosis- relatively mild emotional disorders (such as mild depression and phobias) Neurotoxins- chemicals that attack and damage nerve cells

Neurotransmitters- chemicals that transfer messages from one nerve cell to another or from a nerve cell to a muscle cell

Neutrophil- a type of white blood cell

Nevus- a marking on the skin; can be present at birth (birthmark) or develop later (such as a mole)

Newborn respiratory distress syndrome- a disorder in which premature babies lack surfactant, a substance that stops the lungs from collapsing

Niacin- a vitamin important in many chemical processes in the body; also known as vitamin B3

Night terrors- a form of nightmlare causing abrupt awakening in terror; occurs mostly in children

Nitrates- a group of drugs that widen blood vessels; used to treat insufficient blood supply to the heart (angina pectoris) and reduced pumping efficiency of the heart (heart failure)

Nocturia- urination or a sleep-disturbing need to urinate during the night

Nocturnal emission- ejaculation of semen during sleep, which is normal in adolescent males; commonly called a wet dream

Node- a small, rounded tissue mass

Nodule- a small lump of tissue that is usually abnormal; can form under the skin or protrude

Nondisjunction- an error that occurs during the division of sex chromosomes, causing either too much or too little genetic information to be placed in an egg or sperm when it is formed

Non-Hodgkin's lymphoma- any cancer in lymphoid tissue (found mostly in the spleen and lymph glands) that is not Hodgkin's disease

Non-insulin-dependent diabetes- a type of diabetes mellitus that occurs mainly in those over 40 who are overweight; it is usually treated with diet changes and drugs that increase production of insulin by the pancreas (also known as type II diabetes mellitus)

Noninvasive- a term that is used to describe medical procedures that do not enter or penetrate the body; also refers to noncancerous tumors that do not spread to other sections of the body

Nonnarcotic analgesic- a drug that relieves pain by blocking the production of chemicals that stimulate pain-sensing nerves

Nonsteroidal anti-inflammatory drugs- a group of drugs that relieve pain and reduce inflammation

Nootropic- Improve cognitive function, particularly executive functions, memory, creativity, or motivation.

Norepinephrine- a hormone that regulates blood pressure by causing blood vessels to narrow and the heart to beat faster when blood pressure drops

Norwalk virus- a virus that causes acute gastroenteritis

Nose- nariz

Nosocomial infection- an infection acquired in a hospital

NSAID- see Nonsteroidal anti-inflammatory drug

Nucleic acids- substances found in every living organism that provide the instructions for development; includes DNA and RNA

Nucleotide bases- molecules that form nucleic acids

Nucleus- the center or most important point of an object

Numbness- the lack of sensation in a part of the body because of interruption of nerve impulses

Nurse-midwife- a registered nurse who specializes in the care of a mother and child during pregnancy, labor, and delivery

Nutrient- any substance that the body can use to maintain its health

Nystagmus- persistent, rapid, involuntary movement of the eyes

O

Oat cell carcinoma- another term for small-cell carcinoma

Obesity- a condition in which there is an excess of body fat; used to describe those who weigh at least 20 percent more than the maximum amount considered normal for their age, sex, and height

Obsessive-compulsive disorder- a mental disorder in which a person is obsessed with certain thoughts, leading them to repeatedly perform specific acts; for example, constantly washing the hands out of fear of germs and dirt

Obstructive sleep apnea- the blockage of the airways during sleep, which causes breathing to stop for very short periods of time, commonly caused by excessive relaxation of muscles at the back of the throat

Occlusion- the blocking of an opening or passageway in the body

Occult blood- blood in the feces that can be detected only by chemical tests

Occupational disease- a disease that occurs as a result of factors in the workplace

Occupational therapy- treatment to relearn physical skills lost as a result of an illness or accident

Occupational therapy- Terapia ocupacional

Ocular- describes something related to the eyes

Oculomotor nerves- nerves that stimulate movement of the eyeball

Olfactory nerves- nerves that play a role in the sense of smell

Oligodendroglioma- a rare type of cancerous brain tumor that occurs most commonly in the cerebrum

Oligohydramnios- an unusually small amount of amniotic fluid surrounding the fetus in the uterus, which can lead to complications with the pregnancy

Oligospermia- a low level of sperm in the semen; one of the main causes of infertility in men

Oncogenes- genes that, when altered by environmental factors or viruses, can cause abnormal cell growth

Oocyte- an egg cell that has not developed completely

Oophorectomy- the surgical removal of one or both ovaries; used to treat the growth of ovarian cysts or tumors

Open heart surgery- any operation in which the heart is stopped temporarily and a machine is used to take over its function of pumping blood throughout the body

Ophthalmia- severe inflammation of the eyes
Ophthalmologist- a doctor who specializes in care of the eyes; treats eye diseases and disorders

Ophthalmoplegia- partial or total loss of the ability to move the eyes

Ophthalmoscopy- examination of the inside of the eye using a lighted viewing instrument

Opportunistic infection- infection by organisms that would be harmless to a healthy person, but cause infection in those with a weakened immune system (for example, persons with AIDS or chemotherapy patients)

Optic- pertaining to the eyes

Optician- a person who specializes in the making and adjustment of eyeglasses and contact lenses

Optic nerves- the pair of nerves that carry visual information from the retina to the brain

Optic neuritis- inflammation of the optic nerve, often causing a partial loss of vision

Oral contraceptives- drugs taken in pill form to prevent pregnancy; contain synthetic progesterone and estrogen hormones

Orbit- the socket in the skull that contains the eyeball, along with its blood vessels, nerves, and muscles

Orchiectomy- the surgical removal of one or both of the testicles

Orchiopexy- an operation to correct an undescended testicle

Orchitis- inflammation of a testicle, which can be caused by infection with the mumps virus

Organ donation- an agreement to allow one or more organs to be removed and transplanted into someone else

Organism- any single, functioning form of life

Orgasm- involuntary contraction of genital muscles experienced at the peak of sexual excitement

Orphan drugs- drugs used to treat rare diseases; not normally produced because potential sales are small

Orthopedic therapy- terapia ortopédica

Orthopnea- breathing difficulty experienced while lying flat; can be a symptom of heart failure or asthma

Orthotic- a device used to correct or control deformed bones, muscles, or joints

Osgood-Schlatter disease- painful enlargement and inflammation of the area of the shinbone just below the knee, usually occurring in adolescent boys

Osmosis- the process of passage of the solvent portion of a lesser-concentrated solution through a semipermeable membrane into a higher-concentrated solution until the two solutions are equal in concentration; plays an important role in water distribution in the body

Ossification- the formation and maintenance of bone

Osteitis- inflammation of bone

Osteitis deformans- another name for Paget's disease

Osteoarthritis- see Degenerative arthritis

Osteoarthritis- osteoartritis

Osteoblast- a cell that forms bone

Osteochondritis dissecans- bone degeneration inside of a joint, causing small pieces of bone and cartilage to become detached

Osteochondritis juvenilis- inflammation of a growing section of bone in a child or adolescent

Osteochondroma- a noncancerous tumor made up of bone and cartilage

Osteoclast- a cell that breaks down unwanted bone tissue; also refers to a device for fracturing a bone to correct a deformity

Osteodystrophy- defective bone formation

Osteogenesis imperfecta- a genetic disorder in which bones are abnormally fragile, leading to multiple breaks and deformity

Osteolysis- the softening and destruction of bone

Osteoma- a noncancerous bone tumor

Osteomalacia- the loss of minerals and softening of bones because of a lack of vitamin D; called rickets in children

Osteomyelitis- the inflammation of bones and bone marrow because of an infection, usually caused by bacteria

Osteopetrosis- a rare hereditary disorder in which bones become harder and more dense, causing them to break more easily

Osteophyte- an outgrowth of bone near a joint

Osteoporosis- a condition in which bones become less dense, more brittle, and fracture easily

Osteosarcoma- a cancerous bone tumor

Osteosclerosis- an abnormal increase in density and hardness of bone

Otalgia- the medical term for an earache

OTC remedy- see Over-the-counter remedy

Otitis externa- inflammation of the outer ear due to an infection; commonly called swimmer's ear

Otitis media- inflammation of the middle ear (between the eardrum and inner ear) because of the spread of an infection from the nose, sinuses, and throat

Otorrhea- a discharge from an inflamed ear

Otosclerosis- progressive deafness caused by bone formation around structures in the middle ear

Ototoxicity- harmful effect that some drugs have on the organs or nerves in the ears, which can lead to hearing and balance problems

Outpatient treatment- medical attention that does not include an overnight stay at a hospital

Ovaries- two almond-shaped glands located at the opening of the fallopian tubes on both sides of the uterus; produce eggs and the sex hormones estrogen and progesterone

Overdose- an excessively large dose of a drug, which can lead to coma and death

Over-the-counter remedy- a medication that can be purchased without a physician's prescription

Ovulation- the development and release of the egg from the ovary, which usually occurs halfway through a woman's menstrual cycle

Ovum- another term for an egg cell

Oxidation- a chemical reaction involving active sources of oxygen (called oxygen free radicals) that damages cells

Oximetry- determination of the amount of oxygen in the blood by measuring the amount of light transmitted through an area of skin

Oxygen- a gas that is colorless, odorless, and tasteless; essential to almost all forms of life

Oxygen free radicals- active forms of oxygen found in pollution, cigarette smoke, and radiation that can damage cells and are believed to play a role in the aging process and cancer

Oxytocin- a hormone produced in the pituitary gland that causes contraction of the uterus during childbirth and stimulation of milk flow during breast-feeding

Ozone- a poisonous form of oxygen that is present in the earth's upper atmosphere, where it helps to screen the earth from damaging ultraviolet rays

P

Pacemaker- a small electronic device that is surgically implanted to stimulate the heart muscle to provide a normal heartbeat

Paget's disease- a disorder occurring in the middle-aged and elderly in which bone does not form properly, causing bone weakening, thickening, and deformity

Pain/hurts- dolor / duele

Palate- the roof of the mouth

Palliative treatment- treatment that relieves the symptoms of a disorder without curing it

Pallor- abnormally pale skin; usually refers to the skin of the face

Palpation- the use of the hands to feel parts of the body to check for any abnormalities

Palpitation- an abnormally rapid and strong heartbeat

Palsy- loss of sensation or ability to move

Pancreas- a long gland located behind the stomach that produces enzymes that help to break down food and hormones (insulin and glucagon) that help to regulate glucose levels in the blood

Pancreas- páncreas

Pancreatitis- inflammation of the pancreas, which is often caused by alcohol abuse

Pandemic- a widespread epidemic

Panic disorder- an emotional disorder characterized by attacks of anxiety that have no normal causes; usually made worse by stress

Papilloma- a tumor occurring on the skin or mucous membranes; usually not cancerous

Pap smear- a test in which cells are scraped off the cervix and examined for abnormalities; used to detect changes that might precede cervical cancer and to diagnose viral infections such as herpes simplex

Paracentesis- the insertion of a needle into a body cavity to relieve pressure, inject a drug, or remove a sample for analysis

Paralysis- the inability to use a muscle because of injury to or disease of the nerves leading to the muscle

Paralysis- parálisis

Paramedic- a person trained to give first aid and other emergency medical care

Paranoia- a disorder in which a person becomes overly suspicious and emotionally sensitive

Paraphimosis- strangulation of the head of the penis by a tight or inflamed foreskin that has been pulled back

Paraplegia- complete or partial loss of sensation and movement of the legs

Parasite- an organisms that lives on or in other organisms, from which it obtains nutrients

Parasympathetic nervous system- the part of the autonomic nervous system that is stimulated during times of relaxation

Parathyroidectomy- the surgical removal of one or more of the parathyroid glands

Parathyroid glands- small glands located in the neck that produce a hormone that regulates the levels of calcium in the blood

Parathyroid hormone- a hormone released by the parathyroid glands that plays a role in controlling calcium levels in the blood

Parenteral- the introduction of a substance into the body by any route other than the digestive tract, such as through a vein or muscle

Paresis- partial paralysis

Paresthesia- numbness or tingling in the skin; commonly referred to as "pins and needles"

Parkinson's disease- a brain disorder in which there is a lack of the chemical messenger dopamine, which helps control muscle movement; leads to muscle stiffness, weakness, and trembling

Paronychia- a bacterial or yeast infection of the skin around the nail

Parotid glands- salivary glands located in the mouth near the ears

Paroxysm- a sudden attack or worsening of a disease's symptoms

Partial mastectomy- a treatment for breast cancer in which a tumor is removed, along with the skin covering it and some of the surrounding tissues and muscles

Partial seizure- an abnormal electrical discharge in a certain area of the brain, affecting only certain functions

Passive exercise- exercise of an injured part of the body involving no effort from that injured part

Passive smoking- a nonsmoker inhaling the cigar, cigarette, or pipe smoke of others (called second-hand smoke) in the same area, which increases the nonsmoker's risk of cancer and respiratory disorders

Patella- the medical term for the kneecap

Patent- not obstructed; open

Patent ductus arteriosus- a genetic disorder of the heart in which a channel connecting the pulmonary artery and the aorta fails to close and the heart must work harder to supply the body with blood

Paternity testing- use of blood tests to match up DNA or specific blood proteins to determine whether a man is the father of a child

Pathogen- any substance capable of causing a disease; usually refers to a disease-causing microorganism

Pathogenesis- the production and development of a disease or disorder Pathology- the study of disease

Patient-controlled analgesia- a system for administering pain-killing drugs in which the amount of drug delivered is controlled by the patient

PCR test- The polymerase chain reaction (PCR) is a method widely used to make millions to billions of copies of a specific DNA sample rapidly, allowing scientists to amplify a very small sample of DNA (or a part of it) sufficiently to enable detailed study. PCR was invented in 1983 by American biochemist Kary Mullis at Cetus Corporation. Mullis and biochemist Michael Smith, who had developed other essential ways of <u>manipulating</u> DNA, were jointly awarded the Nobel Prize in Chemistry in 1993

Peak flow measurement- the maximum speed that air is exhaled from the lungs; used to diagnose asthma or to determine the effectiveness of asthma medications

Pectoral muscles- the muscles of the upper part of the chest that move the arm across the body, raise some of the ribs, and move the shoulders

Pellagra- a deficiency of the vitamin niacin; causes dermatitis, diarrhea, and mental disorders

Pelvic examination- an examination of a woman's reproductive organs

Pelvic inflammatory disease- inflammation of a woman's internal reproductive organs, usually as a result of a bacterial infection; one of the most common causes of pelvic pain and infertility in women

Pelvis- the group of bones in the lower part of the trunk that support the upper body and protect the abdominal organs

Penile function tests- tests used to determine the cause of impotence, including blood tests and nerve function tests

Penile implant- an inflatable device surgically inserted into the penis that allows a man with impotence to have sexual intercourse

Penis- the external male reproductive organ, which passes urine and semen out of the body

Pepsin- the enzyme found in gastric juice that helps digest protein

Peptic ulcer- an erosion in the lining of the esophagus, stomach, or small intestine, usually caused in part by the corrosive action of gastric acid

Percolation- A liquid extraction employing gradual descent of water or alcohol through a column of dried plant material, usually powdered, and typically filtered in the process.

Percutaneous- a procedure that is performed through the skin, such as an injection

Perforation- a hole in an organ or body structure caused by disease or injury

Periarteritis nodosa- inflammation and weakening of small and medium arteries

Pericardial effusion- fluid buildup inside of the pericardium, affecting the performance of the heart

Pericarditis- inflammation of the membranous sac that covers the heart, causing chest pain and fever

Pericardium- the membranous sac that covers the heart and the base of the blood vessels that are attached to the heart

Perinatal- occurring just before or just after birth

Periosteum- the tissue covering bones, except the surfaces in joints

Periostitis- inflammation of the periosteum

Peripheral nervous system- the nerves that branch out from the brain and spinal cord to the rest of the body

Peripheral vascular disease- the narrowing of blood vessels in the legs or arms, causing pain and possibly tissue death (gangrene) as a result of a reduced flow of blood to areas supplied by the narrowed vessels

Peristalsis- wavelike movement of smooth muscle-containing tubes, such as the digestive tract

Peritoneum- the membrane that lines the abdominal cavity and covers the abdominal organs

Peritonitis- inflammation of the peritoneum
Pernicious anemia- an anemia caused by a failure to absorb vitamin B12; which is essential in the production of normal red blood cells

Perthes' disease- inflammation of the growing head of a femur; a type of osteochondritis juvenilis

Pertussis- a bacterial infection of the respiratory tract characterized by short, convulsive coughs that end in a whoop sound when breath is inhaled (commonly called whooping cough); mainly affects children

Petit mal- a seizure characterized by loss of awareness for brief periods

PET scanning- see Positron emission tomography scanning

Peutz-Jeghers syndrome- a genetic disorder in which there are polyps in the small intestine and brown melanin spots on the lips, mouth, fingers, and toes

pH- a measure of the acidic or basic character of a substance

Phagocyte- an immune system cell that can surround and digest foreign bodies, unwanted cellular material, and microorganisms

Phantom limb- the sensation of a limb after it has been amputated

Pharmacology- the study of medications, including drug development

Pharyngitis- inflammation of the throat (the pharynx), causing sore throat, fever, earache, and swollen glands

Pharynx- the throat; the tube connecting the back of the mouth and nose to the esophagus and windpipe

Phenothiazines- a group of drugs used as antipsychotics, antihistamines, and antiemetics

Phenylketonuria- a hereditary disorder in which the enzyme that converts the amino acid phenylalanine into another amino acid is defective, meaning phenylalanine must be kept out of the diet

Pheochromocytoma- a noncancerous tumor of cells that produce epinephrine and norepinephrine, causing higher levels of these hormones in the blood and an increase in blood pressure

Phimosis- tightness of the foreskin, which prevents it from being moved back over the head of the penis

Phlebitis- inflammation of a vein

Phlebothrombosis- formation of a blood clot in a vein

Phlegm- mucus and other material produced by the lining of the respiratory tract; also called sputum

Phobia- a persisting fear of and desire to avoid something

Phosphates- salts containing phosphorus; essential to some body functions such as the bones and teeth

Phospholipids- fatty substances that make up the membranes surrounding cells

Phosphorus- a mineral that is an important part of structures such as bones, teeth, and membranes in the body; also involved in numerous other chemical reactions

Photocoagulation- tissue destruction using a focused beam of light

Photophobia- an abnormal sensitivity of the eyes to light

Photosensitivity- an abnormal reaction to sunlight, which usually occurs as a rash

Phototherapy- treatment with some form of light

Physical therapy- the treatment of injuries or disorders using physical methods, such as exercise, massage, or the application of heat

Physical therapy / physiotherapy- terapia física / fisioterapia

Physiology- the study of the body's functions

Phytochemicals- chemicals in plants that might help protect against disorders such as cancer

Pica- a desire to eat materials that are not food

Pickwickian syndrome- extreme obesity along with shallow breathing, sleep apnea, excessive sleepiness, and heart failure

PID- see Pelvic inflammatory disease

Pigmentation- the coloration of the skin, hair, and eyes by the pigment melanin

Pinkeye- inflammation of the membrane that covers the white of the eyes and lines the eyelids, causing redness, discomfort, and a discharge; can be caused by infection or allergies

Pinworm- a small parasite worm that can live in the intestines; commonly affects children

Pituitary adenoma- a noncancerous tumor of the pituitary gland

Pituitary gland- a small, round gland located at the base of the brain that releases hormones that control other glands and body processes

Pityriasis alba- a common childhood or adolescent disorder in which there are pale, scaly patches on the skin of the face

Pityriasis rosea- a mild skin condition in which flat, scaly spots occur on the trunk and upper arms

Pivot joint- a joint designed for rotational movement

PKU- see Phenylketonuria

Placebo- a chemically inactive substance given in place of a drug to test how much of a drug's effectiveness can be attributed to a patient's expectations that the drug will have a positive effect

Placebo effect- the positive or negative response to a drug that is caused by a person's expectations of a drug rather than the drug itself

Placenta- an organ formed in the uterus during pregnancy that links the blood of the mother to the blood of the fetus; provides the fetus with nutrients and removes waste

Placental abruption- the separation of the placenta from the wall of the uterus before childbirth, which causes severe bleeding that threatens the life of the mother and the fetus

Placental insufficiency- a disorder occurring during pregnancy in which the placenta does not function properly, causing the fetus to be deprived of nutrients

Placenta previa- a disorder in which the placenta develops at the lower section of the uterus (close to or covering the cervix); varies in severity, from no effect on a pregnancy to vaginal bleeding and danger to the mother and the fetus

Plague- a serious infectious disease transmitted to humans through bites of rodent fleas

Plantar reflex- the normal curling of the toes downward when the sole of the foot is stroked

Plantar wart- a rough-surfaced, hard spot on the sole of the foot that is caused by a virus

Plaque- an area of buildup of fat deposits in an artery, causing narrowing of the artery and possibly heart disease; dental plaque refers to a coating on the teeth, consisting of saliva, bacteria, and food debris, which causes tooth decay

Plasma- the liquid part of the blood, containing substances such as nutrients, salts, and proteins

Plasma cell- a white blood cell that makes antibodies

Plasmapheresis- a procedure for removing unwanted substances from the blood in which blood is drawn, its plasma is separated and replaced, and the cleansed blood is returned to the body

Platelet- the smallest particle found in the blood, which plays a major role in forming blood clots

Pleura- the double-layered membrane that lines the lungs and chest cavity and allows for lung movement during breathing

Pleural effusion- a buildup of fluid between the membranes that line the lungs and chest cavity (the pleura); causes compression of the lungs, which leads to breathing difficulty

Pleural membranes- the pleura

Pleural rub- a rubbing sound produced by inflamed pleural membranes that can be heard when breathing

Pleural space- the space between the two layers of the pleura

Pleurisy- inflammation of the lining of the lungs and chest cavity, usually caused by a lung infection; characterized by sharp chest pain

Pleurodynia- pain in the chest caused by a virus

Plummer-Vinson syndrome- difficulty swallowing due to an abnormal web of tissue across the upper part of the esophagus

PMS- see Premenstrual syndrome

Pneumoconiosis- a respiratory disease caused by dust inhalation

Pneumocystis pneumonia- an opportunistic infection of the lungs caused by a single- celled parasite

Pneumonectomy- surgical removal of a lung

Pneumonia- inflammation of the lungs due to a bacterial or viral infection, which causes fever, shortness of breath, and the coughing up of phlegm

Pneumonia- neumonía

Pneumothorax- a condition in which air enters the space between the chest wall and the lungs, causing chest pain and shortness of breath; may occur spontaneously or be the result of a disease or an accident

Poisoning- envenenamiento

Poliomyelitis- an infectious disease caused by a virus; usually causes only mild symptoms but in rare cases can attack the brain and spinal cord and cause paralysis or death

Polyarthritis- arthritis occurring in more than one joint

Polycystic kidney disease- a condition in which there are multiple, slow-growing cysts on both kidneys

Polycystic ovary syndrome- a hereditary disease characterized by multiple cysts on the

ovaries, obesity, excessive hairiness, infertility, and irregular menstruation

Polycythemia- an increased amount of red blood cells in the blood

Polydactyly- the presence of an excessive number of fingers or toes

Polydipsia- excessive thirst

Polymyalgia rheumatica- a rare disease of the elderly, characterized by muscle stiffness and pain in the hips, thighs, shoulders, and neck

Polymyositis- an autoimmune disease of connective tissue in which muscles weaken and become inflamed

Polyp- a growth that occurs on mucous membranes such as those in the nose and intestine; bleeds easily and can become cancerous

Polysaccharide- a complex carbohydrate composed of three or more simple carbohydrate molecules joined together

Polyunsaturated fat- a fat or oil that contains well below the maximum number of hydrogen atoms possible; thought to reduce the risk of coronary heart disease

Polyuria- the excessive production of urine; can be a symptom of various diseases, most notably diabetes mellitus

Porphyria- a group of genetic disorders in which substances called porphyrins build up in the blood, often causing rashes brought on by exposure to sunlight and reactions to certain drugs

Portal hypertension- increased blood pressure in the portal vein

Portal vein- the vein connecting the stomach, intestines, and spleen to the liver

Positron emission tomography scanning- an imaging method in which substances emitting positrons (positively charged particles) are introduced into the body, and detectors connected to a computer are used to form images of the tissues

Postcoital contraception- the prevention of pregnancy after sexual intercourse has occurred

Posterior- describes something that is located in or relates to the back of the body

Postmenopausal bleeding- bleeding from the vagina that occurs after menopause

Postmortem examination- examination of a body after death to determine the cause of death; commonly called an autopsy

Postmyocardial infarction syndrome- a condition that occurs following a heart attack or heart surgery; characterized by fever, chest pain, pericarditis, and pleurisy

Postnatal- describes something that occurs after birth, usually to the baby

Postpartum- a term that describes something that occurs after childbirth, usually to the mother

Post-traumatic stress disorder- feelings of anxiety experienced after a particularly frightening or stressful event, which include recurring dreams, difficulty sleeping, and a feeling of isolation

Postural drainage- drainage of mucus from specific areas of the lungs by placing the body in a specific position

Postural hypotension- unusually low blood pressure that occurs after suddenly standing or sitting up

Potassium- a mineral that plays an important role in the body, helping to maintain water balance, normal heart rhythm, conduction of nerve impulses, and muscle contraction

Poultice- A topical preparation typically containing plant solids such as powder or leaves, mashed with water and applied to the skin.

Precancerous- describes a condition from which cancer is likely to develop

Precordial movement- movement of the heart that is seen and felt through the chest wall

Preeclampsia- a serious disorder that occurs in the second half of pregnancy, in which a woman experiences high blood pressure, fluid retention, nausea, and headaches; if not treated it can lead to eclampsia

Premature labor- labor that begins before the full term of pregnancy (about 37 weeks) Premature rupture of membranes- the rupture of the sac that holds the fluid surrounding the fetus before the full term of pregnancy (about 37 weeks)

Premedication- drugs, usually painkillers, taken 1 to 2 hours before surgery

Premenopausal- a term that describes the period of a few years in a woman's life just before menopause

Premenstrual syndrome- physical and emotional changes that occur in a woman 1 or 2 weeks before menstruation, at or after ovulation; characterized by irritability, tension, depression, and fatigue

Prenatal care- medical care of a pregnant woman and the fetus Prenatal diagnosis- techniques used to diagnose abnormalities in a fetus

Prenatal testing- tests performed on a pregnant woman or her fetus to prevent or diagnose abnormalities

Prepared childbirth- a technique in which a pregnant woman tries to minimize use of pain-relief medications during childbirth by learning relaxation techniques

Prepuce- the foreskin

Presbycusis- the loss of hearing that occurs naturally with age

Presbyopia- the loss of the ability to focus the eyes on near objects that occurs naturally with age, as a result of loss of elasticity of the lens of the eyes

Pressure point- specific points on the body where external pressure can be applied to prevent excessive arterial bleeding

Pressure sore- an ulcer (erosion) on the skin that is a result of being bedridden; commonly called a bedsore

Priapism- a painful, persistent erection without sexual arousal, requiring emergency treatment

Prickly heat- a rash involving small, red, itchy spots and a prickly sensation that usually appears where sweat builds up

Primary- a disease that began in the affected location

Prion- an agent that is believed to cause several degenerative brain diseases

Procidentia- severe prolapse of an organ

Proctalgia- pain in the rectum

Proctitis- inflammation of the rectum, which causes soreness and sometimes mucus and/or pus in the stool

Proctoscopy- examination of the rectum using a viewing instrument

Productive cough- a cough that brings up phlegm, which is the body's natural way of clearing blocked airways

Progeria- an extremely rare condition in which the body ages prematurely

Progesterone- a female sex hormone that plays many important roles in reproduction, including the thickening of the lining of the uterus during the menstrual cycle; and during pregnancy, the functioning of the placenta, and the initiation of labor

Prognosis- a doctor's probable forecast of the effects and outcome of a disease Progressive muscular atrophy- gradual degeneration and weakening of muscles due to a degenerative spinal cord

Prolactin- a hormone released by the pituitary gland that is responsible for the development of breasts and milk production in females

Prolapse- the displacement of an organ from its normal position to a new one

Prolapsed disk- see Disk prolapse

Prophylactic- anything used to prevent disease

Proprioception- the body's system for determining its position relative to the outside world

Prostatectomy- the partial or complete surgical removal of the prostate gland

Prostate gland- an organ located under the bladder that produces a large part of the semen

Prostatism- symptoms caused by an enlarged prostate gland, including difficulty with urination

Prostatitis- inflammation of the prostate gland, usually due to a bacterial infection spread from the urethra

Prosthesis- an artificial replacement for a missing part of the body

Proteins- large molecules made up of amino acids that play many major roles in the body, including forming the basis of body structures such as skin and hair, and important chemicals such as enzymes and hormones

Prothrombin time- the time it takes for a sample of blood to clot after substances that speed clotting time have been added; used to measure the effect of anticoagulants

Proton pump inhibitor- a drug used to treat peptic ulcers that reduces the amount of gastric acid produced

Proto-oncogene- a gene that is normally inactive but can become a cancer-causing oncogene if made active

Protozoan- a simple, single-celled organism

Proximal- located nearer to a central point of reference on the body, such as the trunk

Pruritus- the medical term for itching

Pseudogout- a form of arthritis with symptoms similar to gout that results from the depositing of calcium salts in a joint

Pseudomembranous enterocolitis- severe inflammation of the colon as a result of antibiotic use by an immunocompromised individual

Psittacosis- a chlamydial infection resembling influenza that is spread to humans by the droppings of infected birds

Psoralens- drugs that contain chemicals derived from plants; used to treat the skin disorders psoriasis and vitiligo

Psoriasis- a skin disorder characterized by patches of thick, red skin often covered by silvery scales

Psoriatic arthritis- a form of arthritis that develops as a complication of the skin disorder psoriasis

Psychogenic- resulting from psychological or emotional disorders

Psychological- relating to the mind and the processes of the mind

Psychosis- a mental disorder in which a serious inability to think, perceive, and judge clearly causes loss of touch with reality

Psychosomatic- describes a physical condition that is influenced by psychological or emotional factors

Psychotherapy- the treatment of mental and emotional disorders using psychological methods, such as counseling, instead of physical means

Psychotic- relating to psychosis

Psychotropic drug- a drug that has a psychological effect

Ptosis- the drooping of the upper eyelid

Puberty- the period of time (usually between the ages of 10 and 15) during which sexual development occurs, allowing reproduction to become possible

Pubic louse- a small insect that lives in pubic hair, feeds on blood, and is usually spread by sexual contact; pubic lice are popularly called "crabs"

Pudendal block- a local anesthesia procedure used during childbirth, causing the lower part of the vagina to be insensitive to pain

Pudendum- the external genitals, usually referring to the female

Puerperal sepsis- infection of the female genital tract following childbirth, abortion, or miscarriage

Puerperium- the time period after childbirth (about 6 weeks) during which a woman's body returns to its normal physical state

Pulmonary artery- the artery that supplies the lungs with blood from the heart

Pulmonary edema- the buildup of fluid in lung tissue, which is usually caused by heart failure

Pulmonary embolism- blockage of the pulmonary artery by a floating mass in the blood

Pulmonary fibrosis- a condition in which the tissue of the lungs has become thick and scarred, usually because of inflammation caused by lung conditions such as pneumonia or tuberculosis

Pulmonary heart valve- the heart valve that stops blood pumped to the lungs from leaking back into the heart

Pulmonary hypertension- increased blood pressure in the arteries supplying blood to the lungs; caused by increased resistance to blood flow in the lungs, usually a result of a lung disease

Pulmonary insufficiency- a rare defect in the pulmonary heart valve in which it fails to close properly after each muscle contraction, allowing blood to leak back into the heart; weakens the heart's pumping ability

Pulmonary stenosis- obstruction of the flow of blood from the heart to the lungs

Pulp- the soft tissue inside of a tooth that contains blood vessels and nerves

Pulse- the expansion and contraction of a blood vessel due to the blood pumped through it; determined as the number of expansions per minute

Pupil- the opening at the center of the iris in the eye that constricts (contracts) and dilates (widens) in response to light

Purpuric rash- areas of purple or reddish-brown spots on the skin, which are caused by bleeding from underlying tissues

Pus- a thick, yellowish or greenish fluid that contains dead white blood cells, tissues, and bacteria; occurs at the site of a bacterial infection

Pustule- a small blister containing pus

PUVA- a form of phototherapy that combines the use of psoralens and ultraviolet light to treat skin disorders

Pyelolithotomy- surgical removal of a kidney stone

Pyelonephritis- inflammation of the kidney, usually due to a bacterial infection

Pyloric sphincter- a circular muscle located at the junction of the stomach and small intestine that controls the passage of food into the small intestine

Pyloric stenosis- narrowing of the outlet located at the junction of the stomach and small intestine

Pyloroplasty- surgical widening of the outlet between the stomach and small intestine

Pyrexia- a body temperature of above 98.6°F in the mouth or 99.8°F in the rectum

Pyrogen- any substance that causes a fever

Pyuria- the presence of white blood cells in the urine; usually an indication of kidney or urinary tract infection

Q

Quadriceps muscle- the muscle (consisting of 4 distinct parts) located at the front of the thigh that straightens the leg

R

Rabies- an infectious viral disease primarily affecting animals; can be transmitted to humans through an infected animal's bite; if untreated, can result in paralysis and death

Radial keratotomy- a surgical procedure for correcting nearsightedness in which tiny cuts are made in the cornea to change its shape and focusing properties

Radiation- a variety of types of energy, such as X-rays and ultraviolet

Radiation therapy- treatment of a disease, such as cancer, using forms of radioactivity that damage or destroy abnormal cells

Radical surgery- treatment of disease by surgically removing all tissue that is or may be affected

Radiculopathy- any disease of the nerve roots; can be caused by disk prolapse, arthritis, and other problems

Radioallergosorbent test- a blood test performed to help determine the cause of an allergy by detecting the presence of antibodies to various allergens

Radiography- the formation of images of the inside of the body using radiation projected through the body and onto film; a radiograph is also called an X-ray

Radionuclide scanning- an imaging technique in which a radioactive substance is introduced into the body and its emitted radiation is detected; specific organs can be studied according to the amount of the radioactive substance that they absorb

Radius- one of the two long bones of the forearm, located on the thumb side of the arm

Radon- a colorless, odorless, tasteless radioactive gas that is produced by materials in soil, rocks, and building materials; suspected of causing cancer

Rales- abnormal crackling or bubbling sounds heard in the lungs during breathing

Rape kit- In the 1970s, after the women's movement had gained its first traction, The kit was developed in Chicago, to provide a more uniform protocol for evidence collection after sexual assaults. A rape kit consists of small boxes, microscope slides and plastic bags for collecting and storing evidence such as clothing fibers, hairs, saliva, blood, semen or body fluid.

Rash- an area of inflammation or a group of spots on the skin

Rash- sarpullido / erupción

Raynaud's disease- a condition in which the fingers and toes become pale when exposed to cold or emotional stress, owing to sudden narrowing of the arteries that supply them with blood

Receptor- a nerve cell that responds to a stimulus and produces a nerve impulse; also refers to the area on the surface of a cell that a chemical must bind to in order to have its effect

Recessive gene- a gene that does not produce its effect when it occurs with a dominant gene, but produces its effect only when there are two copies of it

Reconstructive surgery- surgery to rebuild part of the body that has been damaged or defective from birth

Rectal exam- A rectal examination is where a doctor or nurse uses their finger to check for any problems inside your bottom (rectum), sometimes ask you to squeeze around their finger so they can assess how well the muscles are working (pause no chakra),

Rectal prolapse- bulging of the lining of the rectum through the anus, usually due to straining during a bowel movement

Rectum- a short tube located at the end of the large intestine, which connects the intestine to the anus

Red blood cell- a doughnut-shaped blood cell that carries oxygen from the lungs to body tissues

Reduction of fracture- the realignment of the broken ends of a bone

Referred pain- pain felt in a part of the body remote from the site where pain originates

Reflex- an automatic, involuntary response of the nervous system to a stimulus

Reflux esophagitis- the backflow of gastric acid from the stomach to the lower esophagus, owing to a defect in the valve that separates them

Regurgitation- the backflow of fluid; can refer to food and drink flowing back up from the stomach into the mouth or blood flowing back into the heart through a defective heart valve

Rehabilitation- treatment for an injury or illness aimed at restoring physical abilities

Rehydration- treatment for dehydration (an abnormally low level of water in the body) in which levels are restored by taking fluids containing water, salt, and glucose by mouth or, if severe, through a vein

Reiter's syndrome- a disorder characterized by inflammation of the joints, urethra, and sometimes the conjunctiva

Relapse- the return of a disease or symptom after it had disappeared

Remission- the temporary disappearance of a disease or its symptoms, either partially or completely; also refers to the time period in which this occurs

REM sleep- rapid eye movement sleep; the stage of sleep in which dreaming occurs

Renal cell carcinoma- the most common type of kidney cancer

Renal colic- severe pain on one side of the lower back, usually as a result of a kidney stone

Renal tubular acidosis- inability of the kidneys to remove sufficient amounts of acid from the body, making the blood more acidic than normal

Renin- an enzyme that plays a role in increasing a low blood pressure

Repetitive strain injury- an injury that occurs when the same movement is repeated continuously

Reproductive system- the organs and structures that allow men and women to have sexual intercourse and produce children

Resection- partial or complete surgical removal of a diseased organ or structure

Respiration- the process by which oxygen is taken in and used by tissues in the body and carbon dioxide is released

Respirator- another term for a ventilator

Respiratory arrest- a condition in which a person suddenly stops breathing

Respiratory distress syndrome- a condition experienced after an illness or injury damages the lungs, causing severe breathing difficulty and resulting in a life-threatening lack of oxygen in the blood

Respiratory failure- the failure of the body to exchange gases properly, which leads to a buildup of carbon dioxide and a lack of oxygen in the blood

Respiratory system- the organs that carry out the process of respiration

Respiratory therapy- terapia respiratoria

Resting pulse- the pulse rate when a person is not experiencing any physical activity or mental stress

Reticulocyte- an immature red blood cell

Retina- a membrane lining the inside of the back of the eye that contains light-sensitive nerve cells that convert focused light into nerve impulses, making vision possible

Retinal artery occlusion- obstruction of an artery that supplies blood to the retina, resulting in some degree of temporary or permanent blindness

Retinitis pigmentosa- gradual loss of the field of vision, owing to a degeneration of the light-sensitive nerve cells of the retina

Retinoblastoma- a hereditary, cancerous tumor of the retina affecting infants and children

Retinoid- a substance resembling vitamin A that is used to treat skin conditions such as acne and has been reported to reduce skin wrinkling

Retinopathy- any disease or disorder of the retina; usually refers to damage to the retina caused by high blood pressure or diabetes mellitus

Retinoscopy- a method of determining focusing errors of the eye in which light is shined through the pupil and the reflected beam is measured

Retroviruses- a group of viruses that are made up of RNA instead of DNA, including HIV and the virus that causes T-cell leukemia

Reye's syndrome- a rare disorder mainly affecting those under the age of 15 that is characterized by brain and liver damage following a viral infection such as chickenpox or the flu; may be linked to taking aspirin to treat a viral infection

Rh blood group- a blood group classifying whether the substances called Rhesus (Rh) factors are present on the surface of red blood cells; the "positive" or "negative" designation in blood classification (for example, "O negative")

Rheumatic fever- a disorder that follows a throat infection by the streptococcus bacteria and causes inflammation in body tissues

Rheumatoid arthritis- a condition in which joints in the body become inflamed, stiff, painful, and sometimes deformed because of the body's own immune system attacking the tissues

Rheumatoid factors- antibodies that are present in about 80% of people with rheumatoid arthritis; their detection through blood testing can help to diagnose the disorder

Rh immunoglobulin- a substance used to prevent a woman who is Rh incompatible with her fetus from becoming Rh sensitized

Rh incompatibility- a condition in which a pregnant woman's Rh factor does not match that of the fetus; can lead to the production of antibodies by the mother that destroy the fetus' red blood cells

Rhinitis- inflammation of the mucous membrane lining the nose, which can cause sneezing, runny nose, congestion, and pain; when caused by substances in the air, it is called allergic rhinitis or hay fever

Rhinophyma- a bulb-shaped deformity and redness of the nose as a result of severe rosacea

Rhinoplasty- surgery that changes the structure of the nose, either to improve appearance or to correct a deformity or injury

Rh sensitized- a condition in which a woman who has a negative Rh factor develops permanent antibodies against Rh-positive blood as a result of exposure to the blood of her fetus; can cause fetal hemolysis in subsequent pregnancies

Rhythm method- a method of preventing pregnancy in which a couple does not have sexual intercourse during the days of the menstrual cycle during which fertilization can occur

Riboflavin- a vitamin belonging to the vitamin B complex that is important in many processes in the body and helps to maintain healthy skin

Rickets- a childhood disease in which bones lack calcium and are deformed as a result of vitamin D deficiency (vitamin D helps the body absorb calcium)

Rigor mortis- the stiffness that occurs in the body after death

Ringworm- a skin infection caused by a fungus that spreads out in an even circle, characterized by ring-like, scaly patches of red skin

Rinne's test- a test that uses a tuning fork to diagnose hearing loss resulting from poor conduction of sound from the outer to the inner ear

RNA- ribonucleic acid, which helps to decode and process the information contained in DNA

Rocky mountain spotted fever- a rare disease transmitted to humans through the bites of ticks; characterized by small pink spots on the wrists and ankles that spread to other parts of the body, become larger, and bleed

Rosacea- a skin disorder that is characterized by patches of red skin on the nose and cheeks and acne-like bumps; most commonly occurs in middle-aged women

Roseola infantum- a common disease in young children characterized by a sudden fever and rash

Rotator cuff- a structure made up of four muscle tendons that reinforces the shoulder joint

Roundworm- a group of worms that includes many of the major human parasites

Rubefacient- Promotes dilation of capillaries near the surface of the skin, therefore promoting local circulation to bring fresh blood supply to the skin, soothing inflammation or congestion.

Rubella- a mild viral infection (also known as German measles) that produces a rash and fever; dangerous when it infects a woman during the early stages of pregnancy, when it can spread causing birth defects in the fetus

Rubeola- another term for measles

Rupture- a tear or break in an organ or tissue

S

Saccharides- a group of carbohydrates, including sugars and starches

Sacroiliac joints - the pair of joints located in the pelvis between the sacrum and the hipbones

Sacroiliitis- inflammation of the sacroiliac joints, which causes pain in the lower body

Sacrum- the triangular bone located at the bottom of the spine that is connected to the tailbone, the hipbones near the sacroilial joints, and the rest of the spine

SADS- see Seasonal affective disorder syndrome

Safe sex- measures taken to reduce the risk of acquiring a sexually transmitted disease, such as the use of a condom

Saline- a salt solution or any substance that contains salt

Salivary glands- a group of glands that secrete saliva into the mouth

Salmonella- a group of bacteria; includes a species that causes food poisoning and another responsible for typhoid fever

Salmonellosis- infection by salmonella bacteria

Salpingectomy- surgical removal of one or both fallopian tubes

Salpingitis- inflammation of a fallopian tube

Salpingography- X-ray examination of the fallopian tubes

Salpingolysis- removal of abnormal scar tissue between a fallopian tube and nearby tissue

Salpingo-oophorectomy- the surgical removal of one or both of the fallopian tubes and one or both of the ovaries

Salpingostomy- surgical opening of a fallopian tube for drainage or removal of an obstruction

Salve- Semi-solid fatty herbal mixture typically applied externally. Common components are primarily an oil and a wax, such as extra virgin olive oil infused with herbs and combined with melted beeswax.

Sarcoidosis- a rare disease with no known cause that leads to inflammation in tissues throughout the body, including the lymph nodes, lungs, liver, skin, and eyes

Sarcoma- a cancer in connective tissue, fibrous tissue, or blood vessels

Saturated fat- fats that contain the maximum amount of hydrogen possible, such as those found in meats and dairy products; can contribute to coronary heart disease and the development of some cancers

Saturday night palsy- temporary paralysis of the arm after extended pressure on a nerve in the armpit

Scabies- a highly contagious skin disorder caused by a mite that burrows into the skin and produces an intense, itchy rash

Scarlet fever- an infectious childhood disease, caused by a streptococcus bacteria, that leads to a sore throat, fever, and rash

Schistosomiasis- infestation by a parasitic blood worm that can damage the liver, bladder, and intestines

Schizophrenia- a group of mental disorders characterized by abnormal thoughts, moods, and actions; sufferers have a distorted sense of reality, and a split personality (thoughts do not logically fit together)

Schönlein-Henoch purpura- inflammation and leakage of blood vessels, causing a rash

Sciatica- pain along the sciatic nerve, which runs down the length of the leg to the foot; usually caused by pressure on the nerve due to disk prolapse or a tumor, abscess, or blood clot

Sclera- the tough, white coating that covers and protects the inner structures of the eye

Scleroderma- an immune system disorder of varying degree that can affect many areas of the body

Sclerotherapy- treatment of varicose veins by injection of a solution that destroys them

Scoliosis- a condition in which the spine curves to one side and usually curves toward the opposite side in another section to compensate, producing a characteristic S shape

Screening- the testing of an otherwise healthy person in order to diagnose disorders at an early stage

Scrotum- the sac containing the testicles

Scurvy- a disease caused by a lack of vitamin C, characterized by weakness, bleeding and pain in joints and muscles, bleeding gums, and abnormal bone and tooth growth

Seasonal affective disorder syndrome- a type of depression that seems to be linked to shorter periods of daylight during the fall and winter

Sebaceous cyst- a swelling that occurs under the skin, most commonly on the scalp, face, ears, and genitals; although usually harmless, can grow very large and become painful if infected

Seborrhea- excessive oiliness of the face and scalp

Sebum- the oily, lubricating substance that is secreted by glands in the skin

Secondary- describes a disease or disorder that follows or is caused by another one

Sedatives- a group of drugs that have a calming effect; used to treat anxiety and pain, bring on sleep, and help relax a person before surgery

Seizure- sudden uncontrolled waves of electrical activity in the brain, causing involuntary movement or loss of consciousness

Seizure- convulsión

Selenium- an element needed by the body only in very small amounts that helps maintain tissue elasticity

Semen- fluid released during ejaculation that contains sperm along with fluids produced by the prostate gland and the seminal vesicles

Semen analysis- a procedure in which a semen sample is examined to determine the amount of sperm present, along with their shape and ability to move; commonly used in the treatment of male infertility

Seminal vesicles- two saclike glands in men that produce part of the fluid in semen

Seminiferous tubules- coiled tubes inside of the testicle that are the site of sperm production

Seminoma- a type of testicular cancer that is made up of only a single type of cell

Senile plaques- abnormal deposits of a protein called amyloid in the brain; characteristic of Alzheimer disease

Sensorineural hearing loss- deafness caused by damage to the inner ear or the nerve that conducts signals from the ear to the brain

Sensory nerve- nerves that carry information about the body's senses toward the brain

Sensory organ- an organ that receives and relays information about the body's senses to the brain

Sepsis- the infection of a wound or tissue with bacteria, causing the spread of the bacteria into the bloodstream; now also known as systemic inflammatory response syndrome caused by a microbe

Sepsis- sepsis / septicemia

Septal defect- a birth defect in which a hole is present in the wall that separates the left and right sides of the heart

Septic arthritis- joint inflammation caused by a bacterial infection

Septicemia- a life-threatening condition in which bacteria multiply in the blood and produce toxic materials; commonly known as blood poisoning; now also known as systemic inflammatory response syndrome.

Septic shock- a life-threatening condition in which tissues become damaged and blood pressure drops due to bacteria multiplying and producing poisons in the blood

Serotonin- a chemical that transmits nerve impulses in the brain, causes blood vessels to constrict (narrow) at sites of bleeding, and stimulates smooth muscle movement in the intestines

Serum- the clear, watery fluid that separates from clotted blood

Sex chromosomes- the X and Y chromosomes that determine a person's gender; women normally have two X chromosomes and men normally have one X and one Y

Sex hormones- hormones responsible for producing sex characteristics and controlling sexual functions

Sex-linked disorder- a disorder that is caused by genes located on the sex chromosomes

Sexually transmitted disease- infections that are most commonly spread through sexual intercourse or genital contact

Shigellosis- a bacterial infection of the intestines, causing abdominal pain and diarrhea

Shingles- a nerve infection caused by the chickenpox virus, causing areas of painful rash covered with blisters

Shin splints- pain and tenderness experienced in the lower leg as a result of damage or strain to leg muscles and tendons; usually caused by exercise

Shock- a reduced flow of blood throughout the body, usually caused by severe bleeding or a weak heart; without treatment, can lead to a collapse, coma, and death

Shoulder- hombro

Shunt- an artificially constructed or an abnormal passage connecting two usually separate structures in the body

Sialogogue- Promotes salivation.

Sickle cell anemia- a genetic disorder in which the red blood cells are abnormal and deformed, causing anemia (reduced ability to transport oxygen in the blood) and clogging of blood vessels; bouts of fever, headache, and weakness result

Sickle cell trait- a less serious form of sickle cell anemia

Sick sinus syndrome- abnormal functioning of the structure that regulates the heartbeat, causing episodes of abnormal heart rhythm

SIDS- see Sudden infant death syndrome

Sigmoidoscopy- an examination of the rectum and the lowest part of the large intestine using a flexible viewing tube inserted through the anus

Silicone- a group of compounds of silicon and oxygen; commonly used as implants in cosmetic surgery because they resist body fluids and are not rejected by the body

Silicosis- a respiratory disease caused by inhalation of dust containing the mineral silica

Single photon emission computed tomography- an imaging technique in which a radioactive substance is introduced into the body and the radiation emitted by the substance is detected by a camera and is transformed into cross-sectional images by a computer

Sinoatrial node- the structure that regulates the heartbeat; a natural "pacemaker" Sinus- a cavity within bone or a channel that contains blood; also refers to an abnormal tract in the body

Sinus bradycardia- a regular heart rate of less than 60 beats per minute

Sinusitis- inflammation of the lining of the cavities in the bone surrounding the nose (the sinuses), usually as a result of a bacterial infection spreading from the nose

Sinus rhythm- normal heart rhythm

Sinus tachycardia- a regular heart rate of over 100 beats per minute

Sjögren's syndrome- a condition characterized by dryness of the eyes, mouth, and vagina that tends to occur along with certain disorders of the immune system

Skin graft- a method of treating damaged or lost skin in which a piece of skin is taken from another area of the body and transplanted in a damaged or missing section

Skin patch- a sticky patch attached to the surface of the skin that releases drugs into the bloodstream

Skin patch test- a diagnostic test in which different allergens are taped to the skin to determine which causes an allergic reaction

Skin prick test- a test performed to determine a person's sensitivity to a certain allergen by applying it to a small needle and using that needle to pierce the skin

Skull- the bones that form the framework of the head and enclose and protect the brain and other sensory organs

Sleep apnea- a condition in which breathing stops for very short periods of time during sleep

Sleeping sickness- an infectious disease in Africa spread by the bite of a tsetse fly that causes a fever and weakness

Slipped disk- the common term for disk prolapse Small-cell carcinoma- the most serious form of lung cancer

Small intestine- the long tube running from the stomach to the large intestine that is involved in digestion of foods and absorption of nutrients

Small intestine- intestino delgado

Smallpox- a highly contagious and often fatal viral infection that has been completely eradicated by immunization

Smear- a sample of cells spread across a glass slide to be examined through a microscope

Smoking- fumar

Sodium- a mineral that plays a role in the body's water balance, heart rhythm, nerve impulses, and muscle contraction; present in table salt (sodium chloride)

Sodium bicarbonate- a substance used as an antacid

Solar plexus- the largest network of nerves in the body, located behind the stomach

Somatic- pertaining to the body

Sore throat- dolor de garganta

Spasm- an involuntary muscle contraction; can sometimes be powerful and painful

Spasticity- muscle stiffness caused by an increase in contractions of the muscle fibers

Spastic paralysis- spasticity involving partial paralysis

SPECT- see Single photon emission computed tomography

Speculum- an instrument that holds an opening of the body open so that an examination can be performed or a sample can be taken

Speech therapy- treatment to help someone overcome a problem communicating verbally Sperm- the male sex cell produced in the testicles

Sperm antibody- an antibody against sperm that can be produced by a woman's immune system

Spermatocele- a harmless cyst containing fluid and sperm that occurs in the tube through which sperm travel from the testicles

Sperm count- the amount of normally functioning sperm per some unit of semen; used to determine a man's fertility

Spermicide- a contraceptive substance that kills sperm

Sphincter- a ring of muscle fibers located around a naturally occurring passage or opening in the body that opens and closes to regulate passage of substances

Sphygmomanometer- an instrument used to measure blood pressure

Spider nevus- a collection of dilated (widened) capillaries on the skin that creates a patch resembling a spider

Spina bifida- a birth defect in which a section of the baby's spine fails to develop completely, leaving the spinal cord exposed in that section

Spina bifida occulta- the least dangerous form of spina bifida, in which bones in the spine fail to close but there is no protrusion of the spinal cord or its fluid cushion out of the body

Spinal cord- a long tube of nerve tissue inside the spinal column, running from the brain down the length of the back inside of the spine

Spinal fusion- the surgical joining of two or more adjacent vertebrae using bone fragments; used to help severe back pain or prevent damage to the spinal cord

Spinal tap- another term for a lumbar puncture

Spine- the column of bones and cartilage running along the midline of the back that surrounds and protects the spinal cord and supports the head

Spiral fracture- a coiled break in a bone, resembling a corkscrew

Spirometry- a test of lung condition; a person breathes into a machine called a spirometer that measures the volume of air exhaled

Spleen- an organ located in the upper left abdomen behind the ribs that removes and destroys old red blood cells and helps fight infection

Splenectomy- surgical removal of the spleen

Splint- a device that is used to immobilize a part of the body

Splinter hemorrhage- a splinter-shaped area of bleeding under a fingernail or toenail

Spondylitis- inflammation of the joints between the bones of the spine

Spondylolisthesis- the slipping of a vertebra in the spine over the one below it

Spondylolysis- a disorder in which the lower part of the spine is weakened by an abnormally soft vertebra

Sporotrichosis- an infection with a fungus acquired through a skin wound; causes an ulcer at the site of infection and small, rounded masses of tissue near it

Sprain- the tearing or stretching of the ligaments in a joint, characterized by pain, swelling, and an inability to move the joint

Sprue- a digestive disorder in which nutrients cannot be properly absorbed from food, causing weakness and loss of weight

Sputum- mucus and other material produced by the lining of the respiratory tract; also called phlegm

Squamous cell carcinoma- a type of skin cancer arising from flat cells of the epithelium; can also affect the lungs, cervix, and esophagus

Stapedectomy- surgical removal of a stapes (a sound-conducting bone in the middle ear) that cannot move to transmit sound; performed to treat hearing loss caused by otosclerosis

Staphylococci- common bacteria that cause skin infections and a number of other disorders

Status asthmaticus- a life-threatening asthma attack requiring immediate treatment

Status epilepticus- a life-threatening succession of epileptic seizures

STD- see Sexually transmitted disease

Stein-Leventhal syndrome- see Polycystic ovary syndrome

Stem cells- cells that give rise to the different types of blood cells

Stenosis- narrowing of a body passageway

Stent- a device used to hold tissues in place, such as to support a skin graft

Stereotaxic surgery- brain surgery done through a small opening in the skull and guided by X-rays or computer-aided imaging techniques

Sterilization- a surgery performed to make a person incapable of reproducing; also refers to the process of killing microorganisms on objects such as surgical instruments

Sternum- the long, flat bone located at the center of the chest

Steroids- a group of drugs that includes corticosteroids, which resemble hormones produced by the adrenal glands, and anabolic steroids, which are similar to the hormones produced by the male sex organs

Stillbirth- a baby that is born dead after the 28th week of pregnancy; also called late fetal death

Stroke- accidente cerebral

Stoma- a surgically formed opening on a body surface

Stomach- estómago

Stomach bypass- a surgical procedure to treat an obstructed stomach or severe obesity in which the passage of food is diverted around the stomach and directly into the small intestine

Stomach stapling- a procedure in which the stomach is made smaller by partitioning it off using metal staples; used as an extreme treatment of severe obesity

Stomachache- dolor de estómago

Stool- another term for feces

Strabismus- a condition in which the eyes are not aligned correctly, such as cross-eye (one eye points inward) and walleye (one eye points outward)

Straight-leg raising- a simple test performed in a doctor's office to check for disk prolapse

Strain- muscle damage resulting from excessive stretching or forceful contraction

Strangulated hernia- a hernia in which the protruding organ or tissue loses its blood supply, requiring emergency surgery

Strawberry nevus- a bright red, raised birthmark that usually disappears without treatment

Strep throat- a throat infection caused by streptococcus bacteria; characterized by a sore throat, fever, and enlarged lymph nodes in the neck

Streptococci- bacteria that cause a variety of diseases, including pneumonia and strep throat

Stress fracture- a bone break resulting from repeated pressure on the bone

Stretch marks- lines on the skin that occur when the inner skin layer is stretched thin and loses its elasticity

Stroke- damage to part of the brain because of a lack of blood supply (due to a blockage in an artery) or the rupturing of a blood vessel; leads to complete or partial loss of function in the area of the body that is controlled by the damaged part of the brain

Stye- a pus-filled abscess in the follicle of an eyelash; caused by a bacterial infection

Subcutaneous- a medical term meaning "beneath the skin"

Submucosa- the layer of connective tissue under a mucous membrane

Suction lipectomy- see Liposuction

Sudden infant death syndrome- the unexpected, sudden death of an apparently healthy baby, the cause of which cannot be found; also called crib death

Sudorific- Promotes sweating

Suppository- a solid cone or bullet-shaped object made up of a chemically inactive substance and a drug that is inserted into the rectum or vagina; used to administer a drug

Suppuration- the production of pus

Surfactant- a mixture of substances secreted by the air sacs of the lungs that prevents the air sacs from collapsing during exhalation

Surrogate- a woman who agrees to become pregnant and give her baby to someone else when the child is born

Suture- a surgical stitch that helps close an incision or wound so that it can heal properly

Sweat glands- tiny structures in the skin that secrete sweat

Sweat test- a measure of the saltiness of sweat to help diagnose cystic fibrosis

Swimmer's ear- see Otitis externa

Sycosis barbae- a bacterial infection of the hair follicles in the beard area

Sympathetic nervous system- the part of the autonomic nervous system that raises blood pressure and heart rate in response to stress

Syndactyly- a condition in which fingers or toes are fused together

Syndrome- a group of symptoms that indicate a certain disorder when they occur together

Synovectomy- surgical removal of the synovial membrane

Synovial fluid- a lubricating fluid secreted by the synovial membrane

Synovial membrane- the thin membrane that lines the inside of a joint capsule

Synovitus- inflammation of the membrane lining a joint capsule as a result of injury or infection or due to a chronic illness such as rheumatoid arthritis; characterized by redness, swelling, stiffness, and pain

Syphilis- a sexually transmitted disease; initially causes only painless sores on the genitals but can be life-threatening if untreated

Syrup- Preparation made by combining a concentrated decoction with either honey or sugar.

Systemic- affecting the whole body

Systemic inflammatory response syndrome- a condition characterized by having two of the following four clinical criteria: fever, rapid breathing, increased heart rate, and abnormal white blood cell count

Systemic lupus erythematosus- a disease of the immune system that causes inflammation of connective tissue in many areas of the body, including the skin, lungs, heart, joints, and kidneys

Systolic pressure- the blood pressure measured while the heart is contracting

Systemic therapy- terapia sistémica

T

Tachycardia- a rapid heart rate (over 100 beats per minute)

Tapeworm- a parasitic worm that lives in the intestines; causes diarrhea and abdominal discomfort

Tar- the sticky, brown substance in cigarettes that coats the lungs; causes lung and other cancers

Tarsorrhaphy- a procedure in which the eyelids are sewn shut; performed to protect the corneas

Tartar- the hard deposit formed on teeth when mineral salts in saliva combine with plaque; can cause dental problems such as gum disease if not controlled

Tay-Sachs disease- a severe genetic disorder that causes nervous system disturbances and death, usually before the age of 3

TB- see Tuberculosis

T cell- see T-lymphocyte

T-cell leukemia- a type of leukemia caused by a virus in which T-lymphocytes divide uncontrollably

Tear duct- a tiny passageway that drains lubricating tears from the surface of the eye to the back of the nose

Telangiectasia- redness of an area of skin, caused by enlargement and proliferation of the underlying small blood vessels

Temperature method- a natural method of family planning in which a woman determines her time of ovulation by changes in her daily temperature

Temporal arteritis- inflammation and narrowing of arteries in the head and neck, including those in the scalp near the temple, which can cause blindness if untreated

Temporomandibular joint syndrome- headache, facial pain, and jaw tenderness caused by irregularities in the way the joints, muscles, and ligaments in the jaw work together

Tendinitis- inflammation of a tendon, usually caused by injury, characterized by pain, tenderness, and sometimes limited movement in the attached muscle

Tendon- strong connective tissue cords that attach muscle to bone or muscle to muscle

Tendon transfer- surgical cutting and repositioning of a tendon so that the muscle attached to it has a new function

Tennis elbow- a form of tendinitis that causes pain and tenderness in the elbow and forearm

Tenosynovitis- inflammation of the inner lining of the sheath that covers a tendon

Tenovaginitis- inflammation of the fibrous wall of the sheath that covers a tendon

TENS- see Transcutaneous electrical nerve stimulation

Tension headache- a headache caused by emotional strain or tension in the muscles of the head and neck

Teratogen- anything that causes abnormalities in a developing embryo or fetus, such as a drug or virus

Teratoma- a tumor composed of cells not normally found in the part of the body when the tumor occurred

Termination of pregnancy- see Abortion

Testicles- the two male sex organs that produce sperm and the sex hormone testosterone

Testicular feminization factor- a genetic disorder in which an individual who is genetically male has the external appearance of a female because the body is unresponsive to testosterone

Testicular torsion- severe pain and swelling of a testicle, due to twisting of the spermatic cord

Testosterone- the sex hormone that stimulates development of male sex characteristics and bone and muscle growth; produced by the testicles and in small amounts by the ovaries

Tetanus- a sometimes fatal disease affecting the brain and spinal cord; caused by infection with bacterium present in soil and manure

Tetracyclines- a group of antibiotic drugs used to treat a wide variety of infections, including bronchitis and some types of pneumonia

Tetralogy of Fallot- a genetic heart disease involving four structural defects in the heart, which result in insufficient levels of oxygen in the blood

Thalamus- a structure in the brain that relays and processes incoming sensory information from the eyes and ears and from pressure and pain receptors

Thalassemia- a group of genetic blood disorders characterized by a defect in the ability to produce hemoglobin, leading to the rupturing of red blood cells (called hemolytic anemia)

Thallium scanning- a type of radionuclide scanning used to assess the heart

Therapeutic range- the range of doses of a drug that will produce beneficial results without side effects

Thoracoscopy- examination of the membranes covering the lungs using an endoscope

Thoracotomy- a procedure in which the chest is surgically opened to operate on an organ in the chest cavity

Thorax- the chest

Thrill- a vibration felt when the hand is placed flat on the chest; caused by abnormal blood flow through the heart as a result of disease

Thrombectomy- removal of a blood clot

Thrombocytopenic purpura- a decrease in the number of platelets in the blood, causing abnormal bleeding of blood vessels into the skin

Thromboembolism- blockage of a blood vessel by a blood clot fragment that has broken off and traveled from another area of the body

Thrombophlebitis- inflammation of a vein, along with clot formation in the affected area

Thrombosis- a condition in which a blood clot (thrombus) has formed inside a blood vessel

Thrombosis- trombosis

Thrombus- a blood clot in a blood vessel

Thrush- a candidiasis infection

Thymoma- a tumor of the thymus gland

Thymus gland- an immune system gland located in the upper part of the chest that plays an important role in the production of T-lymphocytes

Thyroglossal cyst- a swelling at the front of the neck; forms from a duct that fails to disappear during embryonic development

Thyroid gland- a gland located in the front of the neck below the voice box that plays an important role in metabolism (the chemical processes in the body) and growth; the gland produces thyroid hormone

Thyroiditis- inflammation of the thyroid gland

Thyrotoxicosis- a toxic condition resulting from overactivity of the thyroid gland

Thyroxin- a hormone produced by the thyroid gland that helps regulate energy production in the body

TIA- see Transient ischemic attack

Tibia- the thicker of the two long bones in the lower leg; commonly called the shin

Tic- an involuntary, repetitive movement such as a twitch

Tic douloureux- see Trigeminal neuralgia

Ticks- small, eight-legged animals that can attach to humans and animals and feed on blood; sometimes spread infectious organisms via their bites

Tietze's syndrome- inflammation of the cartilage that joins ribs to the breastbone, causing chest pain

Tinea- a group of common infections occurring on the skin, hair, and nails that are caused by a fungus; commonly referred to as ringworm

Tinnitus- a persistent ringing or buzzing sound in the ear

Tipped uterus- an abnormal condition in which the uterus is tilted backward instead of slightly forward

Tissue plasminogen activator- a substance produced by the body and as a genetically engineered drug to prevent abnormal blood clotting

Tissue typing- tests used to determine the compatibility of tissues used in grafts and transplants

T-lymphocyte- a type of white blood cell that fights infections and destroys abnormal cells directly; as compared with releasing antibodies to fight infection

T-lymphocyte killer cell- a type of T-lymphocyte white blood cell that attaches to abnormal cells and releases chemicals that destroy them

TMJ syndrome- see Temporomandibular joint syndrome

Toe- dedo (del pie)

Tolerance- decreased sensitivity of the body to a certain drug, usually either because the liver becomes more efficient at breaking down the drug or the body's tissues become less sensitive to it; increased tolerance creates a need for a higher dose of the drug in order to have the same effects

Tonic- This term is used in a variety of culturally dependent ways. It can mean to strengthen and enliven a specific organ or the whole body. In TCM it typically refers to nutritive therapies whereas in Western Herbalism it traditionally (Eclectic physicians a century ago) refers to therapies that promote elimination and reduce excess.

Tonometry- the procedure used to measure the pressure within the eye; is useful in detecting glaucoma

Tonsillectomy- surgical removal of the tonsils, usually to treat tonsillitis

Tonsillitis- infection and inflammation of the tonsils

Tonsils- masses of lymphoid tissue located at either side of the back of the throat

Tourette's syndrome- a movement disorder characterized by involuntary tics and noises, and in some cases uncontrollable shouting of obscenities

Tourniquet- a device placed tightly around an arm or leg in order to stop blood flow; can be used to locate veins in order to take a blood sample or to control blood flow during some operations

Toxemia- the presence of bacterial toxins in the blood

Toxic epidermal necrolysis- a severe rash in which the outer layers of skin blister and peel off

Toxicity- the extent to which a substance is poisonous

Toxic shock syndrome- a life-threatening condition caused by a staphylococci toxin

Toxin- a poisonous substance

Toxocariasis- human infestation with the larvae of a worm found in the intestines of dogs

Toxoplasmosis- a common protozoan infection that is usually only dangerous to a fetus in early pregnancy or a person who is immunocompromised

TPA- see Tissue plasminogen activator

Trachea- the tube running from the larynx (the voice box) down the neck and into the upper part of the chest, where it divides to form the two bronchi of the lungs; commonly called the windpipe

Tracheitis- inflammation of the trachea

Tracheotomy- insertion of a tube through a surgical opening in the trachea to maintain an open airway

Trachoma- a persistent, contagious form of conjunctivitis that can lead to complications such as blindness if untreated

Traction- the use of tension to hold a body part in place or to correct or prevent an alignment problem

Traditional Chinese Medicine (TCM)- Based on a foundation of over 2,500 years of observation and practice, in the 1950s a myriad of widely used traditional practices were unified by the Chinese government, officially named Traditional Chinese Medicine (TCM), and promoted as a system to be integrated with modern medicine. TCM describes a balance of energetics in terms of yin and yang and a vital force, Qi. The goal of TCM is to correct underlying imbalance and manifestation of illness in a person as opposed to treating a disease. In addition to herbs and food, TCM includes acupuncture, acupressure, massage, and movement therapy (American Botanical Council, 2016).

Transcutaneous- through the skin

Transcutaneous electrical nerve stimulation- a method of relieving pain by applying tiny electrical impulses to nerve endings beneath the skin

Transferrin- a substance in the blood that transports iron throughout the body

Transient ischemic attack- a temporary block in the supply of blood to the brain, resulting in temporary loss of sensation, movement, vision, or speech; often called mini- strokes and can be precursors to a real stroke

Transmissible- able to be passed from one organism to another

Transplant- transferring a healthy tissue or organ to replace a damaged tissue or organ; also refers to the tissue or organ transplanted

Transurethral prostatectomy- removal of cancerous tissue from the prostate gland using a resectoscope (a long, narrow instrument passed up the urethra), which allows the surgeon to simultaneously view the prostate and cut away the cancerous tissue

Trauma- physical injury or emotional shock
Travelers' diarrhea- diarrhea when traveling in a foreign country, caused by contaminated food or water

Tremor- an involuntary, rhythmic, shaking movement caused by alternating contraction and relaxation of muscles; can be the normal result of age or the abnormal effect of a disorder

Triage- a system used to classify sick or injured people according to the severity of their conditions

Trichiasis- growth of the eyelashes inward toward the cornea, causing persistent irritation of the eyeball

Trichinosis- infestation by the larvae of the parasitic worm Trichinella spiralis, usually acquired by eating undercooked pork

Trichomoniasis- infection of the vagina by the single-celled parasite Trichomonas vaginilis, which may cause inflammation, itchiness, and discharge from the vagina

Tricuspid valve- the valve located between the two left chambers of the heart (the left atrium and the left ventricle)

Tricyclic antidepressants- drugs used in the treatment of clinical depression

Trigeminal neuralgia- a disorder of the trigeminal nerve (a cranial nerve) that causes brief attacks of severe pain in the lips, cheeks, gums, or chin on one side of the face

Triglyceride- the main form of fat in the blood; determining levels of triglyceride is useful in diagnosing and treating diabetes, high blood pressure, and heart disease

Trimester- one of three periods lasting about 3 months each; the stages into which pregnancy is divided

Triple X syndrome- the presence of an extra X chromosome in a woman, which may cause some degree of mental retardation

Trismus- the medical term for lockjaw

Trisomy- the presence in the cells of three copies of a certain chromosome instead of the normal two copies

Trisomy 21- see Down syndrome

Trophorestorative- A nutritive herb that supports and restores a particular organ or system.

Tubal ligation- a procedure in which the fallopian tubes are cut and tied off; usually a permanent form of sterilization

Tubal pregnancy- a pregnancy that occurs in the fallopian tubes, with a fertilized egg implanting in the tube instead of the uterus; severely painful and can be fatal if not detected and treated

Tuberculin test- skin tests performed to determine previous infection with tuberculosis; can help rule out the possibility of being currently infected with tuberculosis

Tuberculosis- an infectious bacterial disease transmitted through the air that mainly affects the lungs

Tuberous sclerosis- a genetic disorder of the skin and nervous system characterized by epilepsy, mental retardation, and a skin condition resembling acne

Tuboplasty- surgical repair of a damaged fallopian tube to treat infertility

Tumor- an abnormal mass that occurs when cells in a certain area reproduce unchecked; can be cancerous (malignant) or noncancerous (benign)

Tunnel vision- loss of peripheral vision so that only objects directly ahead can be seen; most commonly due to damage caused by increased pressure within the eye (glaucoma)

Turner's syndrome- a genetic disorder in women in which only one X chromosome is present, or both chromosomes are present but one is defective

Tympanic membrane- the medical term for the eardrum
Tympanoplasty- a surgical procedure used to treat hearing loss in which the eardrum or structures in the middle ear are repaired

Typhoid fever- an acute bacterial infection causing fever, headache, abdominal discomfort, and enlargement of the liver and spleen

Typhus- a group of diseases caused by the microorganism rickettsia, spread by the bites of fleas, mites, or ticks; symptoms include headache, fever, rash, and a series of complications if untreated

U

Ulcer- an open sore that occurs on the skin or on a mucous membrane because of the destruction of surface tissue

Ulcerative colitis- a chronic condition in which ulcers occur on the mucous membrane lining of the colon (the end of the large intestine) and the rectum

Ultrasound scanning- an imaging procedure used to examine internal organs in which high-frequency sound waves are passed into the body, reflected back, and used to build an image; also sometimes called sonography

Ultraviolet light- a form of invisible light in sunlight that is responsible for the tanning and burning of skin and can cause cataracts and skin cancer

Umbilical cord- the tubal structure (consisting of two arteries and one vein) that connects the fetus to the placenta, supplying the fetus with oxygen and nutrients and removing some waste products

Umbilical hernia- a condition present at birth in which a part of the baby's intestines bulge through a weak area of the abdominal wall, creating a swelling around the navel

Unconsciousness- a temporary or prolonged loss of awareness of self and of surroundings Undescended testicle- a testicle that has not moved down from the abdomen, where it develops, into the scrotum

Unsaturated fat- a fat or oil found mainly in vegetables; thought to reduce the risk of coronary heart disease

Urea- a waste product of the metabolism of proteins that is formed by the liver and secreted by the kidneys

Uremia- abnormally high levels of waste products such as urea in the blood

Ureters- two tubes that carry urine from the kidneys to the bladder

Urethra- the tube by which urine is released from the bladder

Urethritis- inflammation of the urethra

Urethrocele- a bulging of the urethra into the vagina

Urethrocystitis- inflammation of the urethra and the bladder

Urinalysis- a group of physical and chemical tests done on a sample of urine to check for various disorders, including those of the kidneys and urinary tract

Urinary bladder- vejiga

Urinary diversion- an operation to allow urine passage when the bladder or urethra has become blocked or been removed

Urinary incontinence- the involuntary release of urine because of the inability to control bladder muscles; may occur as a natural part of the aging process or be caused by an injury or disorder

Urinary tract- the structures in the body that are responsible for the production and release of urine, including the kidneys, ureters, bladder, and urethra

Urticaria- an allergic reaction in which itchy white lumps surrounded by areas of inflammation appear on the skin; commonly called "hives"

Uterine prolapse- a condition in which the uterus moves downward into the vagina due to a weakness of the ligaments and muscles that hold the uterus in place

Uterus- the hollow female reproductive organ in which a fertilized egg is implanted and a fetus develops

Uvea- a structure consisting of the colored area of the eye and the middle layer of the eye that contains blood vessels

Uveitis- inflammation of the uvea

V

Vaccination- a form of immunization in which killed or weakened microorganisms are placed into the body, where antibodies against them are developed; if the same types of microorganisms enter the body again, they will be destroyed by the antibodies

Vaccine- a preparation of weakened microorganisms given to create resistance to a certain disease

Vacuum aspiration- removal of the contents of the uterus using a suction device

Vacuum extraction- a technique used to facilitate childbirth using a suction device to help move the baby through the birth canal

Vagina- the muscular passage connecting the uterus with the outside genitals; a component of the female reproductive system

Vaginismus- an involuntary muscle spasm at the opening of the vagina when sexual intercourse is attempted; can be quite painful and may make sexual intercourse nearly impossible

Vaginitis- inflammation of the vagina, which can be the result of infection, aging, a hormone deficiency, or a foreign object (such as a tampon)

Valve- a structure that allows fluid flow in only one direction

Valvotomy- surgical correction of a narrowed heart valve

Valvular heart disease- a heart valve defect

Valvuloplasty- reconstruction or repair of a narrowed heart valve

Varicella- the medical term for chickenpox

Varices- enlarged or twisted blood or lymph vessels

Varicocele- the appearance of varicose veins around the testicles; commonly occurs and is harmless, but may cause discomfort

Varicose veins- enlarged, twisted veins just below the surface of the skin, caused by defective valves in the veins

Variola- another term for smallpox Vascular- pertaining to blood vessels

Vasculitis- inflammation of blood vessels

Vas deferens- a thin tube that stores and transports sperm

Vasectomy- a usually permanent method of sterilization in which the tubes carrying sperm from the testicles (the vas deferens) are cut and tied off; as a result, the semen will no longer contain sperm

Vasoconstriction- narrowing of blood vessels

Vasodilation- widening of blood vessels

Vasovagal attack- a sudden slowing of the heart, causing fainting

VD- see Venereal disease

Vein- a blood vessel that carries blood toward the heart

Venereal disease- any disease that is usually spread through sexual intercourse or genital contact

Venipuncture- piercing of a vein with a hollow needle to inject fluid or withdraw blood Venography- an X-ray procedure for viewing veins

Venom- a poisonous substance produced by certain animals

Ventilation- the process through which oxygen and carbon dioxide are exchanged between the lungs and the air; also refers to the use of a machine to carry out this process in someone who cannot breathe on his or her own

Ventilator- a machine used to take over breathing when a person cannot breathe on his or her own

Ventricle- a small cavity or chamber; there are four ventricles in the brain that circulate cerebrospinal fluid through it, and two in the heart that pump blood throughout the body

Ventricular fibrillation- rapid, irregular contractions of the heart

Ventricular septal defect- a hole in the wall that separates the two lower chambers of the heart (called the ventricles)

Vernix- the thick, greasy substance that covers the skin of a newborn baby

Version- a shift in the position of the fetus inside of the uterus, either occurring naturally or as performed by a doctor to facilitate delivery

Vertebra- any one of the 33 bones that make up the spine

Vertebral arteries- a pair of arteries running up the neck to supply the brain with blood

Vertebrobasilar insufficiency- episodes of dizziness and weakness caused by insufficient blood flow to the brain

Vertex presentation- the usual, head-first presentation of the fetus during delivery

Vertigo- the feeling that one or one's surroundings are spinning

Very low-density lipoprotein- a class of blood proteins, a high level of which is associated with coronary heart disease

Vesicle- a small skin blister, or any sac in the body, that contains fluid

Vestibular glands- two small glands located at the opening of the vagina that secrete a lubricating fluid during sexual stimulation

Villi- the millions of fingerlike projections on the lining of the small intestine that aid in the absorption of food

Viral- a term describing something related to or caused by a virus

Viral infection- infección viral

Viremia- the presence of viruses in the blood

Virilization- the process by which a woman develops male characteristics; caused by overproduction of male sex hormones

Virulence- the relative ability of an organism to cause disease

Virus- the smallest known disease-causing microorganism; viruses are very simple in structure and can only multiply when they are inside the cell of another organism

Virus- Virus

Visual acuity- a measure of the sharpness of a person's vision

Visual field- the area on both sides that can be seen while looking straight ahead

Vision problems- problemas de visión

Vital sign- any sign, such as a pulse, that indicates that a person is alive

Vitamin A- a vitamin essential for normal growth and development of the body (most notably the bones and teeth), protection of mucous membranes from infection, normal vision, and healthy skin and hair

Vitamin B complex- a group of vitamins including thiamine, niacin, riboflavin, pantothenic acid, pyridoxine, biotin, and folic acid; plays a variety of important roles in the body, including in hormone production, metabolism, and functioning of the nerves, muscle, heart, and digestive system

Vitamin B6- a vitamin that plays an important role in the breakdown and use of energy sources, production of red blood cells and antibodies, and normal functioning of the nervous system

Vitamin B12- a vitamin that is essential to the production of DNA (the genetic material in cells) and red blood cells and in the functioning of the nervous system

Vitamin C- a vitamin with many essential roles, including in maintaining healthy bones, teeth, gums, ligaments, and blood vessels and in the immune system's response to infection

Vitamin D- a vitamin that plays a role in the absorption of calcium by the intestines and is essential for healthy bones and teeth

Vitamin E- a vitamin that protects tissues from damage by oxygen free radicals, helps to form red blood cells, maintains the function of enzymes, and maintains cell structure

Vitamin K- a vitamin that is essential for normal blood clotting and the body's absorption of calcium

Vitamins- complex substances that are necessary in small amounts to maintain health and ensure proper development and functioning of the body

Vitiligo- a condition in which patches of skin on the body lose their color; thought to be caused by the immune system attacking the skin tissues, causing the absence of melanin

Vitreous humor- the clear, watery fluid that fills the cavity of the eye behind the lens

VLDL- see Very low-density lipoprotein

Vocal cords- two strips of tissue in the voice box that have the ability to produce sound when air passing through them causes the tissues to vibrate

Volvulus- twisting and obstruction of an area of intestine

Vomit- vómito

Von Willebrand's disease- a genetic disorder characterized by excessive bleeding

V/Q lung scans- images produced by radionuclide scanning of the lungs; used to help diagnose a pulmonary embolism

Vulnerary- Encourages healing of wounds or inflammation.

Vulva- the outer, visible portion of the female genitals

Vulvitis- inflammation of the vulva

Vulvovaginitis- inflammation of the vulva and vagina

W

Walleye- a condition in which one eye turns outward

Wart- a contagious, harmless growth caused by a virus that occurs on the skin or a mucous membrane

Weber's test- a test in which a vibrating tuning fork is held against the forehead to help determine the cause of hearing loss

Wegener's granulomatosis- a disorder in which nodules associated with inflammation of blood vessels develop in the lungs, kidneys, and nasal passageways

Weight-bearing exercise- exercise that puts stress on bones, such as walking, which helps build up bone density and prevent the bones from becoming brittle

Weight loss- pérdida de peso

Wernicke's encephalopathy- a brain disorder characterized by abnormal eye movements, difficulties with muscle coordination, and confusion; usually the result of chronic alcoholism

Western Herbalism- As one of the modern practices of herbalism in English-speaking Western world (Wood, 2006), traditional Western Herbalism draws from herbal traditions and plants from across the world and throughout history. Traditional Western herbalism has its roots in Greco-Roman medicine, including the humoral system, while also incorporating aspects of Arabic, Ayurvedic, and Traditional Chinese Medicine. The modern clinical practice of Western Herbalism is also informed by the work of Thomsonian, Eclectic, and Physiomedical botanic physicians of the 18th through early 19th century American Botanical Movement. In addition to these various traditions and centuries of clinical and empirical experience, modern Western herbalism is also informed by modern pharmacological research which studies the potential therapeutic applications of specific constituents found in medicinal plants.

Wheeze- a high-pitched sound produced during breathing because of narrowing of the airways; common sign of asthma

Whiplash injury- injury to the ligaments, joints, and soft tissues of the neck region of the spine because of a sudden, violent jerking motion of the head

Whipple's disease- a rare disorder that has widespread effects on the body, including impaired absorption of nutrients, weight loss, joint pain, and anemia

Whipworm- a small, parasitic worm that can live in the intestines of a human and may cause diarrhea, abdominal pain, and anemia

White blood cell- a group of colorless blood cells that are part of the immune system, helping prevent and fight infection

White blood cell count- the number of white blood cells present in a blood sample; useful in diagnosing and evaluating various diseases and infections

Whitehead- a painless, small, white bump; usually occurs in groups on the nose, cheeks, or around the eyes

Whitlow- an abscess on the end of a finger or a toe that is caused by the herpes simplex virus or a bacterial infection

Whooping cough- see Pertussis

Wilm's tumor- a type of kidney cancer that usually affects children under the age of 5

Wilson's disease- a rare genetic disorder in which copper builds up in the liver and is released into other parts of the body, eventually causing damage to the liver and brain

Withdrawal bleeding- bleeding from the vagina that occurs when hormone levels drop, such as menstruation or the bleeding that occurs at the end of each cycle of the combined oral contraceptive pill

Wrist- muñeca

X

Xanthelasma- fatty deposits around the eyes that are common in elderly people and are associated with high levels of cholesterol in the blood

Xanthine- a bronchodilator drug that is used to treat asthma

Xanthomatosis- a condition in which fatty deposits occur in various parts of the body, possibly leading to atherosclerosis

X chromosome- one of the two sex chromosomes; determines female sex characteristics

Xeroderma pigmentosum- a genetic disorder in which the skin is extremely sensitive to sunlight, causing it to age prematurely and leaving the individual particularly susceptible to skin cancer

Xerophthalmia- excessive dryness of the cornea and conjunctiva due to a lack of vitamin A

X-linked disorder- a genetic disorder in which the abnormal gene is located on the X chromosome; those affected are almost always men

X-ray- see Radiography

XYY syndrome- a disorder in which a man has an extra Y chromosome, causing him to be unusually tall and to have behavioral disorders

Y

Y chromosome- one of the two sex chromosomes; determines male sex characteristics

Yeast infection- a term usually referring to a candidiasis infection

Yellow fever- a life-threatening viral infection transmitted by mosquitoes that causes jaundice, fever, headache, and vomiting

Z

ZIFT- see Zygote intrafallopian transfer

Zinc chloride- a white powder used as an antiseptic and antiperspirant

Zollinger-Ellison syndrome- a rare disorder in which tumors form in the pancreas and secrete the hormone gastrin, which causes increased production of gastric acid and recurrent peptic ulcers

Zoonosis- a parasite-caused or infectious disease in animals that can be transferred to humans

Zygote- the cell that results when an egg is fertilized by a sperm

Zygote intrafallopian transfer- a method used to treat infertility in which an egg fertilized outside the body is placed into a woman's fallopian tube

TECHNOLOGY EQUIPMENT RECAP

Melanocytes - Photovoltaic Cells

Neurons/Nerves - Electromagnetic Cells

Fascia - Plasma Medium (misonomered Ether)

Brain - CPU, Inductor

Brainstem - Two-way Adapter for CPU into the Motherboard

Pineal Gland - Receiver, Crystal Tuner & Actuator Arm/ Head responsible for Phosphorescence, Thermoluminescence, Piezoelectricity, Birefringence & Harmonic Generation (very much like the otoconia in the ears)

Operating System - Deductive Logic or PQ

Heart - Hydraulic Ram, Turbine (from the Greek τύρβη, tyrbē, or Latin turbo, meaning **vortex**) and Hard Drive.

Melanosomes - Alternators

Mitochondria - Motors

Myelin Sheath - Insulation

Cytoskeleton - Filaments

Phospholipids - Capacitors

Spine - Piezoelectric, Motherboard, Radio Wave Antenna

RBC - Floppy Discs

Lymph Nodes - Filters, Nodes

Protein - Transformer

Transformers 'Roll Out' - Conformational Change (Macromolecule Shape Shifting)

Antioxidants - Semi-conductors (especially the selenium based...)

Body Cells - Plasma based Crystal disc, fitted with integrated circuits as well as gates and channels (see Human Cell Membrane and/or Computer Chip)

Nerves & Vessels - 'Copper' wires (CoAxial Cables) and Fiber Optics

Pigment, Nerve & Blood Clusters - Input Devices like a Mouse, Keyboard, etc...

DNA - Piezoelectric, Antenna, Data Storing Inductors.

Collagen Based Tissue - Piezoelectric Inductors

Stomach - Chemical Mixer

Lumen - the SI unit of luminous flux = to the amount of light emitted per second..... or hollow structures in vessels and cells... hmmm????

Eyes - Camera Lens/Charge Coupled Device (CCD), Digital to Analogue Converter, Complex Photovoltaic Cells/ Photodetector...

Amino Acids - Fuses that can be almost anything!

Nucleic Acid - Actual Intelligence (self powering too).

<u>N-Type Semiconductors</u> - Selenium or Silica doped with Phosphorus (Alkaline-ish)

<u>P-Type Semiconductors</u> - Selenium or Silica doped with Boron (Acid-ish)

<u>PN Junction</u> - <u>Crystal Lattice Structure</u> Material allowing the flowing of electrons in one direction.

<u>Bone and Fascia</u> seem to be a massive N-Type, P-Type, PN Junction Super computer on it's own… especially if we add in the Piezoelectricity & Vitamin D!

<u>Melanin</u> - CPU Core, Solar Repeater

<u>Human Cell Membrane and/or Computer Chip</u> - A flat semiconducting (crystal) disc or wafer, with integrated circuits (resistors/conductors) and/or gates & channels. We now have to add the filaments into this Crystal Disc we call a Body Cell or Somatic Cell.

<u>Transistors</u> - a semiconductor device with three connections, capable of amplification in addition to rectification.

The location that a virus goes viral in, is called a **<u>Hotspot</u>**? WTH!

<u>Virus</u> - an infective agent that typically consists of a nucleic acid molecule in a protein coat, is too small to be seen by light microscopy, and is able to multiply only within the living cells of a host.

Wait you see that, it is happening again! Host…

See look there is another definition of **<u>Virus</u>** - a piece of code that is capable of copying itself and typically has a detrimental effect, such as corrupting the system or destroying data.

Wait a damn minute! DNA is a piece of **<u>code</u>**… A viral strand of DNA or RNA that can jump host is fully capable in that context of copying itself, one would even argue, that is it's only 'motion'.

The detrimental effects of corrupting the system (physical illness) or destroying data (mental illness), can clearly be seen anthropomorphically.

Host - an animal or plant on or in which a parasite or commensal organism lives. VS

Host - store (a website or other data) on a server or other computer so that it can be accessed over the internet.

Transmission is the act of transferring something from one spot to another, like a radio or TV broadcast, or a disease going from one person to another.

I am highlighting the unknown and proposing we may have some answers! Infection - an infectious disease.

plural noun: infections "a chest infection"

Vs

Infection - the presence of a virus in, or its introduction into, a computer system. What is a computer system?

Computer System - a computer system is a programmable electronic device that can accept input; store data; and retrieve, process and output information.

Pandemic language = Virology/Biology language. The question is, why? The next question is what does that have to do with Dr. Sebi or Robert Becker? The obvious....

Computer System - a computer system is a programmable electronic device that can accept input; store data; and retrieve, process and output information.

Computer System - a single information processor but usually a group of processors that have specified and general computations; grouped by hardware ie... liver cells, lung cells, brain cells etc.. What you think?

<u>Exercise</u> - activity requiring physical effort, carried out to sustain or improve health and fitness.
"exercise improves your heart and lung power"

<u>Exercise</u> - computer training or computer based training.

<u>Resonance</u> - the quality in a sound of being deep, full, and reverberating. "the resonance of his voice"

- The ability to evoke or suggest images, memories, and emotions."the concepts lose their emotional resonance"

- The reinforcement or prolongation of sound by reflection from a surface or by the synchronous vibration of a neighboring object.

- The condition in which an electric circuit or device produces the largest possible response to an applied oscillating signal, especially when its inductive and its capacitative reactances are balanced.

- The condition in which an object or system is subjected to an oscillating force having a frequency close to its own natural frequency.

- The occurrence of a simple ratio between the periods of revolution of two bodies about a single primary.

- The state attributed to certain molecules of having a structure that cannot adequately be represented by a single structural formula but is a composite of two or more structures of higher energy.

- • A short-lived subatomic particle that is an excited state of a more stable particle.

Induction - the action or process of inducting someone to a position or organization."the league's induction into the Baseball Hall of Fame"

Induction - a formal introduction to a new job or position.plural noun: inductions
"an induction course"
enlistment into military service.

Induction - The process or action of bringing about or giving rise to something."isolation, starvation, and other forms of stress induction" the process of bringing on childbirth or abortion by artificial means, typically by the use of drugs.

Induction - The inference of a general law from particular instances.

Induction -"the admission that laws of nature cannot be established by induction" the production of facts to prove a general statement.

Induction - a means of proving a theorem by showing that if it is true of any particular case it is true of the next case in a series, and then showing that it is indeed true in one particular case.

Induction - noun: mathematical induction; plural noun: mathematicals inductionthe production of an electric or magnetic state by the proximity (without contact) of an electrified or magnetized body.

Induction - The production of an electric current in a conductor by varying the magnetic field applied to the conductor.

Induction - The stage of the working cycle of an internal combustion engine in which the fuel mixture is drawn into the cylinders.

Is there anyone reading this that would disagree with our body fitting these definitions, the definitions of a computer?

Man this thought experiment just got a lot more interesting didn't it? MIT and the US Military are different types of receipts huh? Is it possible frequency resonance, spreads disease? Human modems? Can Shedding be a broadcast signal?

Wi-Fi is a wireless networking technology that uses radio waves to provide wireless high-speed Internet access. A common misconception is that the term **Wi-Fi** is short for "wireless fidelity," however Wi-Fi is a trademarked phrase that refers to IEEE 802.11x standards.

Viral shedding is a term for when viruses are replicating or reproducing, the virus is being led out of the host cell where it's replicating or
reproducing ... Viral shedding is the expulsion and release of virus progeny following successful reproduction during a host cell infection. Once replication has been completed and the host cell is exhausted of all resources in making viral progeny, the viruses may begin to leave the cell by several methods.

Vaccine - a substance used to stimulate immunity to a particular infectious disease or pathogen, typically prepared from
an inactivated or weakened form of the causative agent or from its constituents or products.

Vaccine - a program designed to detect computer viruses and inactivate them.

"the rate of use of vaccines for computer viruses is not as high as in the US, Japan, and other countries"

Application - a medicinal substance put on the skin.

Application - a program or piece of software designed and written to fulfill a particular purpose of the user.

In our thought experiment, if a virus is simply the media for harmful information...

Media - an intermediate layer in the wall of a blood vessel or lymphatic vessel.

Media - the main means of mass communication (broadcasting, publishing, and the internet) regarded collectively.

DOPE - an illicit drug (such as heroin or cocaine) used for its intoxicating or euphoric effects
especially : MARIJUANA (dopamine altering)

Dope - a preparation (such as an anabolic steroid, diuretic, or tranquilizer) given to a racehorse to help or hinder its performance

To Dope - In semiconductor production, to dope is the intentional introduction of impurities into an intrinsic semiconductor for the purpose of modulating its electrical, optical and structural properties. The doped material is referred to as an extrinsic semiconductor.

Short Circuit - Cardiac Arrest?

Short Circuit - Multiple Sclerosis (due to loss of insulation)

Overheating - Fever?

Overcurrent - Inflammation

With Infection and Virus included we are onto something.

Current - belonging to the present time; happening or being used or done now.

Current - *a body of water* or air *moving in a definite direction*, especially *through a surrounding body of water* or air in which there is less movement.

Current - a flow of electricity that results from the ordered directional movement of electrically charged particles.

Current - a quantity representing the rate of flow of electric charge, usually measured in amperes.

Current - the general tendency or course of events or opinion.

Leakage Current - the unintended loss of energy, gain of resistance or results of faulty/worn out insulation.

Plasma - Electric Currents or Electric Current Carrier

Electric Current - Magnetic Field (AtomSphere) Carrier

Alternating Magnetic & Electric Waves - Light

NeuroTransmitters - Record of ElectroMagnetic Waves produced by Neurons (ElectroChemical Message)

Hormones - Large simple versions of NeuroTransmitters (ElectroChemical Message)

Malware - External Negative Mental Programming

Food - Informative Electronic Batteries

Conductor - a person who directs the performance of an orchestra or choir.

Conductor - a material or device that conducts or transmits heat, electricity, or sound, especially when regarded in terms of its capacity to do this.

Lymphatic System - Watermill

Circulatory System - Generator

Integumentary System - Photovoltaic Diaphragm

Immune System - Antivirus, Malware Scanner, Frequency Filter

& Rectifier

Nervous System - Power Transmission and Cellular Communications Lines

Fascia System - HydroElectric Grid

Respiratory System - Windmill

Windmill - a structure that converts wind power or "air" power into rotational energy or vortex energy, to mill grain. In our case grain is Magnetism!

MAGNETS ARE DEFINED BY GRAINS

MAGNETIC GRAINS ARE DEFINED BY APPLIED

STRESS AND CRYSTAL GEOMETRY

SPM SUPERMAGNETIC

SD SINGLE DOMAIN

PSD PSEUDO DOMAIN

MD MULTIDOMAIN

Reproductive System - Quine (self-replicating programs)

Skeletal System - Piezoelectric Crystal Shaped to produced highly specific frequency under stress, Dynamic Oscillators.

Urinary System - Industrial Wastewater, Return Flow, Surface Runoff, Urban Runoff Agricultural & Animal Husbandry Wastewater

Digestive System - Massive Inductor

Endocrine System - Programmer for Human Cell Membrane and/or Crystal Gel Computer Chips

Human Being - Resonator

COMMON COLDS

Rhinovirus

According to the American Lung Association, 10–40% of all colds are caused by a rhinovirus. There are 100 types of rhinoviruses. They are highly contagious but generally very mild.

Coronavirus

There are about six types of seasonal coronaviruses that can infect humans and cause illness.

Most types of coronavirus result in mild to moderate symptoms of respiratory infections known as **severe acute respiratory syndrome (SARS)**.

The best-known type of coronavirus is SARS-CoV-2, which causes **COVID-19**.

HPIV

HPIV is most likely to cause symptoms in young children and older adults, but anyone can become ill if they contract this common virus. Typically, people with HPIV have very similar symptoms to people with colds caused by rhinovirus, such as a sore throat, sneezing, and congestion.

Symptoms of HPIV are often mild and will resolve on their own with rest and over-the-counter (OTC) medication.

Adenovirus

Adenoviruses are another common virus type that can lead to colds. There are about 50 types

Trusted Source
 of adenovirus. In addition to colds, they can lead to more serious infections, including bronchitis and pneumonia.

Adenoviruses can also infect the lining of the eye and are often the virus responsible for conjunctivitis (pink eye).

RSV

RSV is a common virus that is very similar to rhinovirus. It spreads quickly and typically causes mild respiratory symptoms. It's slightly more common in young children and people over 70 years old, but anyone can contract RSV and develop symptoms at any time.

It's possible for RSV to progress to more serious infections, but you can typically treat it at home with rest and OTC medications.

VACCINES

- Adenovirus
- Anthrax
  - AVA (BioThrax)
- Cholera
  - Vaxchora
  -
- <u>Coronavirus</u>
- Diphtheria
  - DTaP (Daptacel, Infanrix)
  - Td (Tenivac, generic)
  - Tdap (Adacel, Boostrix)
  - DTaP-IPV (Kinrix, Quadracel)
  - DTaP-HepB-IPV (Pediarix)
  - DTaP-IPV/Hib (Pentacel)
  - DTaP-IPV-Hib-HepB (Vaxelis)
- Hepatitis A
  - HepA (Havrix, Vaqta)
  - HepA-HepB (Twinrix)
- Hepatitis B
  - HepB (Engerix-B, Recombivax HB, Heplisav-B)
  - DTaP-HepB-IPV (Pediarix)
  - HepA-HepB (Twinrix)
  - DTaP-IPV-Hib-HepB (Vaxelis)
- *Haemophilus influenzae* type b (Hib)
  - Hib (ActHIB, PedvaxHIB, Hiberix)

- DTaP-IPV/Hib (Pentacel)
  - DTaP-IPV-Hib-HepB (Vaxelis)
- Human Papillomavirus (HPV)
  - HPV9 (Gardasil 9) (For scientific papers, the preferred abbreviation is 9vHPV)
- Seasonal Influenza (Flu) only
  - IIV* (Afluria, Fluad, Flublok, Flucelvax, FluLaval, Fluarix, Fluvirin, Fluzone, Fluzone High-Dose, Fluzone Intradermal)
    *There are various acronyms for inactivated flu vaccines – IIV3, IIV4, RIV3, RIV4 and ccIIV4.
  - LAIV (FluMist)
- Japanese Encephalitis
  - JE (Ixiaro)
- Measles
  - MMR (M-M-R II, Priorix)
  - MMRV (ProQuad)
- Meningococcal
  - MenACWY (Menactra, MenQuadfi, Menveo)
  - MenB (Bexsero, Trumenba)
- Mumps
  - MMR (M-M-R II, Priorix)
  - MMRV (ProQuad)
- Pertussis
  - DTaP (Daptacel, Infanrix)
  - Tdap (Adacel, Boostrix)
  - DTaP-IPV (Kinrix, Quadracel)
  - DTaP-HepB-IPV (Pediarix)
  - DTaP-IPV/Hib (Pentacel)
  - DTaP-IPV-Hib-HepB (Vaxelis)
- Pneumococcal
  - PCV13 (Prevnar13)
  - PCV15 (Vaxneuvance)
  - PCV20 (Prevnar20)
  - PPSV23 (Pneumovax 23)
- Polio

- - Polio (Ipol)
  - DTaP-IPV (Kinrix, Quadracel)
  - DTaP-HepB-IPV (Pediarix)
  - DTaP-IPV/Hib (Pentacel)
  - DTaP-IPV-Hib-HepB (Vaxelis)
- Rabies
  - Rabies (Imovax Rabies, RabAvert)
- Rotavirus
  - RV1 (Rotarix)
  - RV5 (RotaTeq)
- Rubella
  - MMR (M-M-R II, Priorix)
  - MMRV (ProQuad)
- Shingles
  - RZV (Shingrix)
- Smallpox
  - Vaccinia (ACAM2000):
- Tetanus
  - DTaP (Daptacel, Infanrix)
  - Td (Tenivac, generic)
  - Tdap (Adacel, Boostrix)
  - DTaP-IPV (Kinrix, Quadracel)
  - DTaP-HepB-IPV (Pediarix)
  - DTaP-IPV/Hib (Pentacel)
  - DTaP-IPV-Hib-HepB (Vaxelis)
- Tuberculosis
- Typhoid Fever
  - Typhoid Oral (Vivotif)
  - Typhoid Polysaccharide (Typhim Vi)
- Varicella
  - VAR (Varivax)
  - MMRV (ProQuad):
- Yellow Fever

- YF (YF-Vax)

IV

IV Fluids

IV fluids are used to quickly repair the Watermill system, we use our liquid mineral solutions from AmericanHealer.Website

The body has different types of water/plasma reserves that all have different mineral, protein, ion, vitamin, etc... concentration... You could say the body is Colloidal.

Basic IV Fluids Ingredients

The 4 common types of IV fluids include:

1. Normal Saline
2. Half Normal Saline
3. Lactated Ringers
4. Dextrose

Osmosis

Is the 'scale' that balances things on the inside and outside of every Cell Membrane. Each cell membrane is an instrument, individually participating in the Weighing of the Heart Ceremony.

By moving molecules (notes on sheet music) into or out of a membrane, we change the charge value.

Water seeks to balance itself out. A dehydrated cell, with low water levels will 'drink' water molecules into it from the extracellular fluid, regulated by the cell membrane. Water molecules, ions, etc... would conversely be pushed of the cell, if the inside of the cell had more water molecules than the outside.

Osmotic Pressure
The water level regulates Osmotic Pressure, this is the magic that keeps the cell Gel from spilling out. This allows the Enqi Cycle to take place and a wide variety of different types of waters/plasmas to coexist.

The Basics of IV Fluids

IV fluids come in either crystalloid or colloid form. Isotonic, hypotonic, or hypertonic, directly affecting what that solution is used for.

Isotonic - denoting or relating to a solution having the same osmotic pressure as some other solution, especially one in a cell or a body fluid.

Hypotonic - having a lower osmotic pressure than a particular fluid, typically a body fluid or intracellular fluid.

Hypertonic - having a higher osmotic pressure than that of a specified, generally physiological, solution.

Why IV Fluids for Dehydration?

Our bodies contain 60-80% water essential to our survival. You're dehydrated when you don't have enough water &/or nutrients in our water for our body. Severe dehydration can occur if you:

- Have diarrhea, sweating, vomiting

- Have overexercised, prolonged heat exposure

- Have serious injury or burns

- Have surgery &/or you have been unconscious

Types of IV Fluids

Crystalloid or colloid, comes in isotonic, hypotonic, or hypertonic, determines when and if each fluid can be used. Crystalloid are the most common of normal saline in most hospitals.

Crystalloids

Normal Saline

Normal saline is also called 9% normal saline, NS, or 0.9NaCL, generally isotonic.

Fluid resuscitation in **extracellular fluid** is the usual use of this type if IV, due to its high effectiveness. Assuming sufficient red blood cell count, IV increases the circulating plasma volume.

Diabetics often need rehydration due to excessive urination and lack of understanding. Saline is the fluid used when giving blood.

To much sodium can cause excess fluid retention or edema, stressing a already weak heart and kidneys, so it must be used with cautioun in patients with diabetic, cardiac or renal complications.

Half Normal Saline

Also called 0.45NaCl or 45% normal saline, half normal saline is widely used.
Half normal saline has 1/2 the chloride concentration of normal saline and is a hypotonic, crystalloid solution of sodium chloride in water.

It's used for things like:

- Raising your fluid volume
- Simple rehydration
- Sodium chloride balance
- Various fluid reserves

Lactated Ringers

An alternative to normal saline, named after the Sydney Ringer, who developed a solution containing sodium, chloride, calcium, and potassium. Alexis Hartmann discovered that adding lactate to the solution made it more suitable for children.

A IV with electrolytes and a buffer (lactate) makes it isotonic.

No magnesium, unlike serum, makes it the closest thing to the body's natural plasma.

Dextrose

There are many variations of sugar IVs.
Dextrose is a type of corn sugar. Chemically identical to glucose it has several uses in a medical setting.
The 3 basic types of dextrose solutions:

- Dextrose in water

- Dextrose in saline

- Dextrose in Lactated Ringer's

Colloids

Colloids have larger molecules, so colloidal solutions cannot cross cell membranes as crystalloid solutions do. Colloid solutions remain intravascular, for the main Watermill reserves. This means they stay in your circulatory system. This is why they are used for plasma resuscitation.

Which IV fluid is best for diabetic patients?

Ringer's lactate. The mineral element concentration is similar to that in human plasma, treatment with balanced crystalloids may lead to a faster recovery from DKA.

There is now a whole variety of athletic and designer IVs, IV Bars etc... this is just the basic lingo...

PREFIX	MEANING	EXAMPLE OF USE IN MEDICAL TERMS
A-, An-	Without; Lacking	Anemia
Andr/o-	Male	Androgen
Anti-	Against	Anticholinergic drugs
Auto-	Self	Autocrine
Bio-	Life	Biology
Chem/o-	Chemistry	Chemotherapy
Contra-	Against	Contraception
Cyt/o-	Cell	Cytokine
Dis-	Separation; Taking apart	Dissection
Dys-	Difficult; Abnormal	Dyspnea
Eu-	Good; Well	Eupnea
Fibr/o-	Fiber	Fibrosis
Gluco-, Glyco-	Glucose; Sugar	Glycogen
Gyn/o-, Gynec-	Female	Gynecology
Hydr/o-	Water	Hydrocephalus
Idio-	Self; One's own	Idiopathic
Lyso-, Lys-	Break down; Destruction; Dissolving	Lysosome
Mal-	Bad; Abnormal	Malignant
Myc/o-	Fungus	Mycetoma

Necr/o-	Death	Necrosis
Neo-	New	Neonate
Oxy-	Sharp; Acute; Oxygen	Oxytocin
Pan-, Pant/o-	All or everywhere	Pancytopenia
Pharmaco-	Drug; Medicine	Pharmacist
Re-	Again; Backward	Rejuvenation
Somat/o-, Somatico-	Body; Bodily	Somatic cell

Body Part Prefixes

PREFIX	MEANING	EXAMPLE OF USE IN MEDICAL TERMS
Acous/o-	Hearing	Acoustic meatus
Aden/o-	Gland	Adenoid
Adip/o-	Fat	Adipocyte
Adren/o-	Gland	Adrenal cortex
Angi/o-	Blood vessel	Angioplasty
Arteri/o-	Artery	Arteriole
Arthr/o-	Joint	Arthroplasty
Bucc/o-	Cheek	Buccal cavity
Bronch/i-	Bronchus	Bronchioles
Burs/o-	Bursa	Bursa
Carcin/o-	Cancer	Basal cell carcinoma
Cardi/o-	Heart	Cardiology
Cephal/o-	Head	Cephalic flexure

Chol-	Bile	Cholesterol
Chondri-	Cartilage	Chondrosarcoma
Coron-	Heart	Coronary arteries
Cost-	Rib	Costal cartilage
Crani/o-	Brain	Cranium
Cutane-	Skin	Cutaneous
Cyst/o-, Cysti-	Bladder or sac	Cystoscopy
Derm-, Dermat/o-	Skin	Dermatologist
Duoden/o-	Duodenum	Duodenitis
Gastr-	Stomach	Gastrectomy
Gloss-	Tongue	Glossectomy
Hem-, Hema-, Hemat-, Hemo-, Hemat/o-	Blood	Hematopoiesis
Hepat/o-, Hepatico-	Liver	Hepatic portal system
Hist/o-, Histio-	Tissue	Histology
Hyster/o-	Uterus	Hysterectomy
Ileo-	Ileum	Ileostomy
Ischi/o-	Ischium	Ischial tuberosity
Kerat/o-	Cornea (eye or skin)	Keratin
Lacrim/o-	Tear (from your eyes)	Lacrimal fluid
Lact/o-, Lacti-	Milk	Lactose
Laryng/o-	Larynx	Laryngitis
Lingu/o-	Tongue	Lingual tonsil
Lip/o-	Fat	Lipolysis
Lymph/o-	Lymph	Lymphocyte
Mamm-, Mast/o-	Breast	Mammary glands
Mening/o-	Meninges	Meningitis
Muscul/o-	Muscle	Musculoskeletal

My/o-	Muscle	Myocardium
Myel/o-	Spinal cord or bone marrow	Myelin
Nephr/o-	Kidney	Nephron
Neur/i-, Neur/o-	Nerve	Neuron
Oculo-	Eye	Oculomotor nerve
Onco-	Tumor; Bulk; Volume	Oncogene
Onych/o-	Fingernail; Toenail	Onychodystrophy
Oo-	Egg; Ovary	Oocyte
Oophor/o-	Ovary	Oophorectomy
Op-, Opt-	Vision	Optic nerve
Ophthalm/o-	Eye	Ophthalmic artery
Orchid/o-, Orchio-	Testis	Orchidectomy
Orth/o-	Straight; Normal; Correct	Orthostatic
Osseo-	Bony	Osseous tissue
Ossi-	Bone	Ossicles
Ost-, Oste/o-	Bone	Osteoporosis
Ot/o-	Ear	Otolaryngologist
Ovar/i-, Ovario-, Ovi-, Ovo-	Ovary	Ovarian follicle
Phalang-	Phalanx	Phalanges
Pharyng/o-	Pharynx; Throat	Pharyngeal tonsil
Phleb/o-	Vein	Phlebotomist
Phren/i-, Phreno-, Phrenico-	Diaphragm	Phrenic nerve
Pleur-, Pleur/a-, Pleur/o-	Rib, **pleura**	Pleural cavity
Pneum/a- Pneumat/o-	Air; Lung	Pneumonia
Proct/o-	Anus; Rectum	Proctoscopy
Prostat-	Prostate	Prostatectomy
Pseudo-	0	Pseudostratified
Psych/o-, Psyche-	Mind	Psychiatrist

Radio-	Radiation; Radius	Radioisotopes
Ren/o-	Kidney	Renal cortex
Retin-	Retina (of the eye)	Retinitis pigmentosa
Rhin/o-	Nose	Rhinoscope
Salping/o-	Tube	Salpingo-oophorectomy
Sarco-	Muscular; Flesh-like	Sarcomere
Schiz/o-	Split; Cleft	Schizophrenia
Sclera-, Sclero-	Hardness	Sclerosis
Sigmoid/o-	Sigmoid colon	Sigmoidoscopy
Sperma-, Spermo-, Spermato-	Sperm	Spermatocyte
Splen/o-	Spleen	Splenomegaly
Sten/o-	Narrowed; Blocked	Stenosis
Stern-	**Sternum**	Sternoclavicular joint
Stom/a-, Stomat/o-	Mouth	Stomatitis
Thorac/o-, Thoracico-	Chest	Thoracic cavity
Thromb/o-	Blood clot	Thrombolytic
Thyr/o-	Thyroid gland	Thyroiditis
Trache/o-	**Trachea**	Trachealis
Tympan/o-	Eardrum	Tympanic membrane
Ur/o-	Urine	Urologist
Vagin-	Vagina	Vaginal
Varic/o-	Duct; Blood vessel	Varicose veins
Vasculo-	Blood vessel	Vasculitis
Ven/o-	Vein	Venae cavae
Vertbr-	Vertebra; Spine	Vertebral column

Color Prefixes

PREFIX	MEANING	EXAMPLE OF USE IN MEDICAL TERMS
Chlor/o-	Green	Chlorophyll
Chrom-, Chromato-	Color	Chromosome
Cyano-	Blue	Cyanosis
Erythr/o-	Red	Erythrocyte
Leuk/o-	White	Leukocyte
Melan/o-	Black	Melanin

PREFIX	MEANING	EXAMPLE OF USE IN MEDICAL TERMS
Cry/o-	Cold	Cryotherapy
Elect-	Electrical activity	Electrocardiogram
Kin/o-, Kine-, Kinesi/o-	Movement	Kinetic energy
Kyphy/o-	Humped	Kyphosis
Rhabd/o-	Rod-shaped; Striated	Rhabdomyosarcoma
Phot/o-	Light	Photoreceptor
Reticul/o-	Net	Reticulocytes
Scoli/o-	Twisted	Scoliosis
Therm/o-	Heat	Thermotherapy

PREFIX	MEANING	EXAMPLE OF USE IN MEDICAL TERMS
Ab-, Abs-	Away from	Abductor
Ad-	Towards	Adductor
Ante-	Before; Forward	Antenatal

Circum-	Around	Circumcision
Cycl-	Circle; Cycle	Cyclic neutropenia
De-	Away from; Ending	Dehydration
Dia-	Across; Through	Diagnosis
Ect/o-, Exo-	Outer; Outside	Exocrine gland
End/o-, Ent-, Enter/o-	Within; Inner	Endocrine gland
Epi-	Upon; Outside of	Epidermis
Ex-, Extra-	Beyond	Expiration
Infra-	Beneath; Below	Infratemporal fossa
Inter-	Between	Interstitial fluid
Intra-	Within	Intracellular fluid
Meso-	Middle	Mesoderm
Meta-	Beyond; Change	Metabolism
Para-	Alongside; Abnormal	Parathyroid glands
Path/o-	Disease	Pathologist
Peri-	Around	Pericardium
Post-	Behind; After	Postpartum
Pre-	Before; In front	Precancerous
Retro-	Backward; Behind	Retroperitoneum
Sub-	Under	Subcutaneous layer
Super-	Above	Superior
Supra-	Above; Upon	Supraglottis
Sy-, Syl-, Sym-, Syn-, Sys-	Together	Syndrome
Trans-	Across; Through	Transdermal

PREFIX	**MEANING**	**EXAMPLE OF USE IN MEDICAL TERMS**

Bi-	Two	Biceps
Brady-	Slow	Bradycardia
Diplo-	Double	Diploid
Hemi-	Half	Hemihypertrophy
Hetero-	Other; Different	Heterogeneous
Homo-	Same	Homozygous genotype
Hyper-	Above; Beyond; Excessive	Hypertension
Hypo-	Under; Deficient	Hypotension
Iso-	Equal; Like	Isointense
Macro-	Large; Long; Big	Macrophage
Mic-, Micro-	Small	Microglia
Mon-, Mono-	One	Monocyte
Olig/o-	Few; Little	Oliguria
Poly-	Many; Excessive	Polyuria
Quadri-	Four	Quadriceps
Semi-	Half	Semilunar valves
Tachy-	Fast	Tachycardia
Tetra-	Four	Tetralogy of Fallot
Tri-	Three	Triceps
Uni-	One	Unicellular

SUFFIX	MEANING	EXAMPLE OF USE IN MEDICAL TERMS
-ac	Pertaining to	Cardiac
-blast, -blasto, -blastic	Bud; Germ	Myeloblast
-cyte, -cytic	Cell	Thrombocyte

-dynia	Pain; Swelling	Thoracodynia
-eal, -ial	Pertaining to	Esophageal
-ectasis	Expansion; Dilation	Atelectasis
-emia	Blood condition	Anemia
-ia	Condition	Hemophilia
-iasis	Condition; Formation of	Psoriasis
-ism	Condition	Hypothyroidism
-ites, -itis	Inflammation	Arthritis
-ity	Pertaining to	Immunity
-ium	Structure or tissue	Epithelium
-lysis, -lytic	Break down; Destruction; Dissolving	Osteolytic
-malacia	Softening	Osteomalacia
-megaly	Enlargement	Acromegaly
-oid	Resembling	Arachnoid trabeculae
-oma	Tumor	Angiosarcoma
-osis	Condition; Usually abnormal	Endometriosis
-ous	Pertaining to	Aqueous
-pathy	Disease	Lymphadenopathy
-penia	Deficiency; Lack of	Thrombocytopenia
-phagia, -phagy	Eating; Swallowing	Dysphagia
-phasia	Speech	Aphasia
-plasia, -plastic	Growth	Hyperplasia
-plegia	Paralysis	Hemiplegia
-pnea	Breathing	Sleep apnea

-poiesis	Production	Hemopoiesis
-ptosis	Falling; Drooping	Apoptosis
-rrhage, -rrhagic	Bleeding	Hemorrhage
-rrhea	Flow or discharge	Diarrhea
-sclerosis	Hardening	Arteriosclerosis
-sis	Condition	Agranulocytosis
-stasis	Level; Unchanging	Homeostasis
-trophy	Growth	Hypertrophy
-uria	In the urine	Anuria

SUFFIX	MEANING	EXAMPLE OF USE IN MEDICAL TERMS
-centesis	Surgical puncture to remove fluid	Thoracentesis
-desis	Surgical binding	Pleurodesis
-ectomy	Cut out; Removal	Mastectomy
-gram	Record; Picture	Electrocardiogram
-graph	Instrument used to create a record or picture	Electrocardiograph
-graphy	To record or take a picture	Echocardiography
-meter	Device used for measuring	Sphygmomanometer
-opsy	Visual examination	Biopsy
-ostomy	Opening	Colostomy
-otomy	Incision	Laparotomy
-pexy	Surgical fixation	Oophoropexy
-plasty	Surgical reconstruction	Vertebroplasty

-scope	For examining	Endoscope
-scopy	Examine	Endoscopy

ENGLISH TERMS	SPANISH TERMS
insulin	insulina
metformin	metformina
ibuprofen	ibuprofeno
aspirin	aspirina
simvastatin	simvastatina
omeprazole	omeprazol
sodium levothyroxine	levotiroxina sódica
ramipril	ramipril
amlodipine	amlodipino
losartan	losartan
enalapril	enalapril
captopril	captopril
paracetamol	paracetamol
acetaminofen	acetaminofen
salbutamol	salbutamol
lansoprazole	lansoprazol
sodium chloride	cloruro de sodio
colecalciferol	colecalciferol

bisoprolol fumarate	bisoprolol fumarato
co-codamol	co-codamol
bendroflumethiazide	bendroflumetiazida
amoxicillin	amoxicilina
azithromycin	azitromicina
amitriptyline hydrochloride	hidrocloruro de amitriptilina
warfarin sodium	warfarina sódica
metamizole	metamizol
codeine	codeína
penicillin	penicilina

The Rectal Examination

Michael J. McFarlane.

A wag once remarked, with considerable truth, that a consultant is a doctor who makes a rectal examination.

—r. h. major, m.d.

Definition

Rectal examination consists of visual inspection of the perianal skin, digital palpation of the rectum, and assessment of neuromuscular function of the perineum.

Technique

The clinical situation and experience of the examiner will often dictate which of several methods to employ in performing the rectal examination. In the lithotomy position, the patient is supine with the legs drawn in toward the trunk and the knees allowed to fall out to the side. This position is customarily used when examining the pelvic organs in women and may offer a better examination of the anterior rectum. The lateral decubitus, or Sim's position, provides optimal examination when the patient is too ill or otherwise unable to assume other positions. The patient lies on the left side with the buttocks near the edge of the examining table or bedside with the right knee and hip in slight flexion. The proctologic (knee–chest or prone jackknife) position is the preferred position in which to examine the perineum and rectum properly. In this position, the patient can easily undergo further studies such as anoscopy and sigmoidoscopy because of easier access to the anorectum. Regardless of the position used, the rectal examination involves both inspection and palpation. First, using a gloved hand, the examiner inspects the buttocks for fistulous tracts, the skin tags of hemorrhoids, excoriations, blood, and rectal prolapse. The patient then is asked to bear down to check again for rectal prolapse and for proper descent of the perineum, the area between the thighs from the coccyx to the pubis. In normal individuals, the perineum lies about 2.5 cm above the ischial tuberosities. When straining at stool, the perineum will descend approximately 1.5 cm or to a level about 1 cm above the ischial tuberosities. Next, the examiner applies firm pressure on the ischial tuberosities in order to evaluate early abscess or fistual formation found in inflammatory bowel disease. With pressure still applied to the perineum, the patient is asked to bear down again in order to obtain further evidence of an abscess or fistula.

The next step of the rectal examination involves the assessment of neuromuscular integrity. First, each side of the buttocks is scratched with the gloved finger to elicit the superficial anal reflex (the anal "wink"), a function of L1 and L2. Next, using a generous amount of water-soluble gel for lubrication, the gloved index finger is inserted gently into the rectum. While the patient consciously acts to resist defecation (analogous to stopping in midstream during urination), the examiner should evaluate the anterior contraction of the puborectalis muscle and the contraction of the external anal sphincter. The patient then relaxes, and the examiner pushes the puborectalis muscle posteriorly, noting the relaxation of the internal anal sphincter. Finally, the patient bears down again, expelling the examining finger, causing the puborectalis muscle to move posteriorly and the internal anal sphincter to relax. This maneuver often permits palpation of the cervix in women and allows assessment of tenderness of this organ.

The final step of the rectal examination assesses anatomic integrity by digital palpation. Once again, the gloved finger is slipped gently into the rectum, and the entire circumference of the rectum is systematically palpated in two stages. The first stage involves the area 1 to 2 cm beyond the external sphincter (the length of the fingerpad), and the second stage deals with the remainder of the rectum within reach of the examining finger, about 7 or 8 cm. Attention should be given to the presence of masses, tenderness, hemorrhoids, fissures, ulcers, and the color and consistency of the stool, with special emphasis on the posterior rectal shelf. In men, the prostate, its size, consistency, and presence of nodules should be noted (see Chapter 192), including assessment of the area of the rectovesicular pouch. In women, the rectouterine pouch of Douglas should be palpated for masses or tenderness. Bimanual examination (rectoabdominal or rectovaginal) often facilitates examination of the lower abdomen and genitourinary structures.

Basic Science

The rectum begins at the termination of the sigmoid colon about 12 cm from the anal verge (Figure 97.1). Two muscle bundles, known as the internal and external anal sphincters, participate in defecation. The internal anal sphincter is an enlargement of the circular smooth muscle of the colon and functions involuntarily. The external anal sphincter consists of striated muscle bands under the voluntary control of the puborectalis muscle. The rectum has the same innervation as the bladder; the hypogastric nerves innervate the internal anal sphincter, and the internal pudendal nerve (S3–S4) operates the external anal sphincter. Because of the common innervation, dysuria is a common complaint associated with rectal disorders.

An important landmark both anatomically and clinically is the pectinate line where the anus and rectum merge, approximately 3 to 4 cm from the skin. It serves as a demarcation for venous and lymphatic drainage and for the nerve supply. Above the pectinate line, the veins drain into the portal and caval systems, sympathetic nerves are present (pain is absent), and lymph drains to the superior rectal and iliac nodes. Below the pectinate line, the veins drain into the caval system alone, innervation is through somatic nerves (pain is present), and lymph drains into the inguinal nodes.

The rectum functions to permit defecation in a voluntary fashion. Peristalsis propels the stool from the sigmoid colon into the rectum. Increased intraluminal pressure causes involuntary relaxation of the internal anal sphincter followed by reflex contraction of the external anal sphincter, preventing incontinence while providing awareness of imminent defecation. The external anal sphincter then relaxes in a voluntary fashion, expelling the feces. Studies suggest that the evacuative process is facilitated by larger fecal bulk, providing an impetus for encouraging patients to consume diets high in fiber and bulk.

Clinical Significance

As Major alluded as long ago as 1937, many otherwise puzzling clinical situations are resolved when a rectal examination is made. Indeed, the history and physical examination are incomplete without the rectal examination; it should not be omitted. Any person with abdominal complaints (e.g., abdominal or rectal pain, diarrhea, constipation, nausea, vomiting, or bleeding) needs a rectal examination to direct further diagnostic and therapeutic maneuvers appropriately. Although disagreement exists as to what age and how often, the American Cancer Society recommends yearly rectal examination and testing for occult blood in the stool for all persons after age 40 as a screening procedure for both colorectal and prostate carcinoma.

Inspection of the buttocks often provides clues to many disorders, including skin tags from hemorrhoids, fistulous tracts, and fissures in patients with inflammatory bowel disease, rectal prolapse, and superficial ulcers caused by herpes simplex or syphilis. The perianal skin may also be affected by generalized disorders including psoriasis and vitiligo or infective processes such as syphilitic dermatitis and candidiasis.

The assessment of neuromuscular function is necessary in

many situations because simple palpation of the external anal sphincter is a poor measure of strength and cannot diagnose dysfunction. Patients with fecal incontinence often complain of "diarrhea" because the anal canal is unable to handle a normal volume of stool, or the sensation of the urge to defecate is inadequate. These individuals often provide a history of traumatic childbirth or surgical repair of hemorrhoids with subsequent disruption of the sphincter musculature or innervation. Upon examination, the descent of the perineum is often much greater than normal, often dropping below the plane of the ischial tuberosities. In addition, fecal incontinence may be the first symptom of serious systemic diseases such as neuropathies, spinal cord tumors (primary or metastatic), or multiple sclerosis.

Palpation of the rectum can reveal ulcers from herpes, syphilis, or inflammatory bowel disease, as well as fistulae or fissures not seen on inspection. Diligent palpation of the rectum should be made to determine the presence of masses because 22% of colorectal cancers arise from the rectum, and this organ may be the site of metastatic disease as well. Masses are not all neoplastic and may be abscesses. Fluctuant consistency of the mass and the presence of fever suggest abscess.

Tenderness is one of the more helpful signs on rectal examination. The location and degree of tenderness may provide additional or convincing evidence of such disorders as prostatitis, pelvic inflammatory disease, tubo-ovarian abscesses, ovarian cysts, ectopic pregnancy, and inflammatory bowel disease. Rectal tenderness in suspected appendicitis has been touted as an important diagnostic clue, but the weight of evidence suggests that this finding is of little help.

The importance of noting the consistency, color, and presence of frank or occult blood in the stool cannot be overemphasized. Elderly patients, with or without a history of chronic constipation, may present with diarrhea that rectal examination will discover to be due to fecal impaction. Black stools result from degraded blood (melena), iron, licorice, bismuth, rhubarb, or overindulgence in chocolate cookies. Red-colored stools may be due to brisk bleeding known as hematochezia (usually distal to the ligament of Treitz), whereas patients under treatment for tuberculosis may complain of red- or orange-colored stools due to rifampin. One of the first symptoms of hepatobiliary disease is the development of tan stools and dark urine. Very rarely, a patient with carcinoma of the ampulla of Vater presents with a complaint of silver stools.

Busy practitioners often omit the rectal examination for a variety of reasons. The procedure allegedly takes too much time, causes discomfort to the patient, and is not aesthetically pleasing. In many diseases, however, examination of the rectum will point the physician in the proper diagnostic direction. This, in turn, may obviate the need for expensive and unnecessary laboratory and/or radiologic evaluation. The diligent, conscientious, and thorough physician will make the rectal examination a necessary part of a complete patient evaluation. An anonymous quote is relevant: "For most diagnoses all that is needed is an ounce of knowledge, an ounce of intelligence, and a pound of thoroughness."